**Books are to be returned on or before
the last date below.**

WITHDRAWN FROM STOCK

WITHDRAWN FROM STOCK

D1348420

Color Atlas of

PERIPHERAL VASCULAR DISEASES

Second Edition

Jill J F Belch MB FRCP MD (Hons)
Professor of Vascular Medicine and Consultant Physician
University Department of Medicine

Peter T McCollum MB MCh FRCSI
Consultant Vascular Surgeon and Honorary Senior Lecturer
University Department of Surgery

Peter A Stonebridge ChM FRCSE
Consultant Vascular Surgeon and Honorary Senior Lecturer
University Department of Surgery

William F Walker DSc ChM FRCS FRCS (Edin) FRS (Edin)
Formerly Professor and Consultant Surgeon
University Department of Surgery
Ninewells Hospital and Medical School
Dundee, Scotland

Mosby-Wolfe

London Baltimore Barcelona Bogotá Boston Buenos Aires Caracas Carlsbad, CA Chicago Madrid Mexico City Milan Naples, FL New York
Philadelphia St. Louis Seoul Singapore Sydney Taipei Tokyo Toronto Wiesbaden

Project Managers	Simon Pritchard, Dave Burin
Development Editor	Lucy Hamilton
Cover Design	Ian Spick
Layout	Simon Pritchard
Illustration Manager	Lynda Payne
Production	Siobhan Egan
Index	Jill Halliday
Publisher	Geoff Greenwood

CONTENTS

PREFACE TO THE SECOND EDITION

The second edition of this colour atlas has involved a careful review and update of contents and a radical redesign. The peer-group response to the first edition reflected an appreciation of a style of book that was both user-friendly and academically stimulating: thus, the format of the book has not been changed.

The need for updating the text, however, arose from the progress made over the past few years in the field of vascular diseases. While atherosclerotic vascular disease in all its various forms still accounts for nearly half of all male deaths in industrialized countries, the techniques used to detect these disorders have changed considerably. Vascular surgery, in particular, has benifitted from new techniques used in the measurement and detection of both macro- and microvascular diseases. Risk factors for the development of vascular disease have also been covered for the first time with reference to hyperlipidaemia, smoking and hypertension. A new section on vascular medicine includes the many microvascular diseases, such as connective tissue diseases and vasculitides.

These changes to the second edition enhance the content of the book, which remains one of the few publications devoted entirely to peripheral vascular diseases

JJFB
PTM
PAS
WFW

PREFACE TO THE FIRST EDITION

Vascular disease in its various forms accounts for nearly half the deaths in the western world and for a considerable loss of work and suffering

Fortunately over the past 30 years there have been rapid developments in our understanding of vascular physiology, pathology, aetiology and therefore to some extent its prevention, clinical presentation and finally treatment. Because the last is continually evolving and changing, only the principles will be discussed here. Particular attention is focussed on visual recognition of the various states as these even in the early stage may be diagnostic.

Vascular disease is not necessarily a disease of one area of the vascular system but is usually widespread with emphasis in a localised area. It is necessary therefore to consider the whole patient since coexistent disease, the presence of diabetes or hyperlipidaemia, or other conditions such as cancer have a considerable effect on prognosis and treatment.

This book presents vascular disease in a pictorial form, It should be a useful supplement to the many detailed and excellent books on vascular surgery.

William F Walker
1980

ACKNOWLEDGEMENTS

We should like to record our indebtedness to our colleagues and friends both here in Dundee and throughout the UK for their help in preparing the slides used in this book. These include the following:

Professor C D Forbes
Dr P D James
Professor K G Lowe
Dr M Nimmel
Dr D G Rushton

Dr J W Shaw
Mr M G Walker
Dr M Wilkinson
Mr R A B Wood

1.

Pathophysiology

Peripheral arterial disease (PAD) is a common disorder producing a significant degree of morbidity in the general population. Atheromatous disease is by far the most common; however, other pathological events can produce similar clinical pictures. These include vasospastic disorders, inflammatory vascular disease, vascular trauma, tumours and congenital malformations.

ATHEROMA

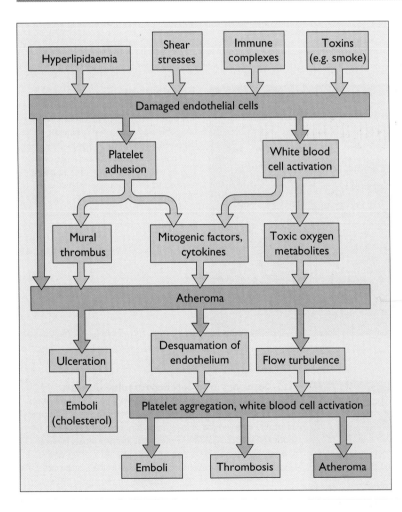

1.1 Development of atheroma.
In the UK, 5% of men over 50 years of age have intermittent claudication, which is the commonest manifestation of atheromatous PAD, and this progresses to critical limb ischaemia (CLI) in 8–12%. The 'response to injury' hypothesis of atherosclerosis development suggests that the initiating factors for atheroma are chemical or mechanical injury. There are many non-mechanical mediators of injury, for example, white blood cells (WBCs) and platelets, as well as wear and tear due to abnormal haemodynamics and flow-mediated stresses. Chemicals released from the endothelium, WBCs and platelets interact and contribute to the proliferation of smooth muscle cells. These effects, in combination with lipid deposition within the macrophage, lay the fatty streak foundation for the development of atheroma.

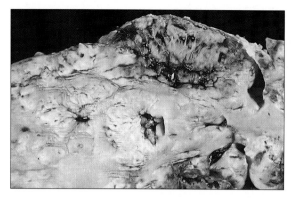

1.2 Fatty streak. The initial lesion in atheroma is the fatty streak, which on microscopic examination shows the presence of lipid-laden foam cells. Initially the lipid is concentrated within cells in the immediate subendothelial region. Later the fat-filled cells may disintegrate, allowing an increase in extracellular lipid deposition. This slide shows the end result (i.e. atheroma).

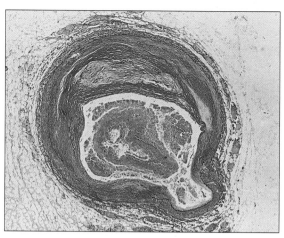

1.3 Subintimal atheroma. This histological section shows narrowing of the artery with subintimal atheroma. The atheromatous plaque shows as a blue–red area at the top of the picture.

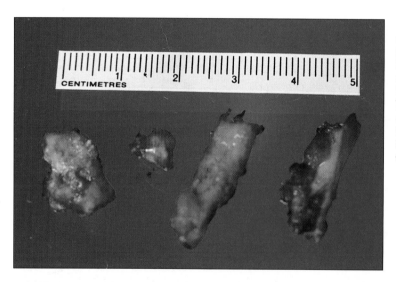

1.4 Atheroma. This 'porridge-like' deposit below the intima is atheroma. In this case, it has become organized and has extended along the artery for some distance, forming an intravascular plug. This can be excised (endarterectomy). This atheromatous material has been excised from a common iliac vessel. On the left, an ulcerated plaque can be seen; on the right, recently formed thrombus.

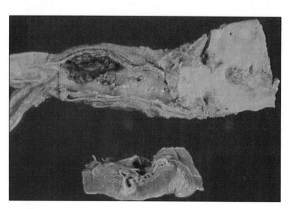

1.5 Coronary and cerebrovascular disease. This is the cause of reduced life expectancy in patients with PAD. Patients with intermittent claudication have a 5% yearly mortality rate, which is 2–3 times higher than expected. In patients with critical limb ischaemia the prognosis is even worse, with a 10–20% annual mortality. At the top of this illustration, severe disease can be seen in the aorta and common iliac arteries. At the bottom, in the same patient, narrowing of a coronary artery is seen with myocardial ischaemic fibrosis in its area of distribution.

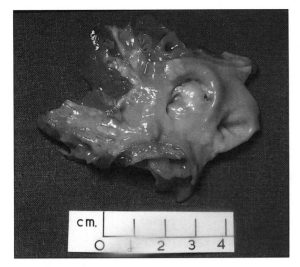

1.6 Mitral stenosis atheroma. Atheroma may even involve the pulmonary artery secondary to pulmonary hypertension due to mitral stenosis, as seen here. The lipoid material is shown as yellow plaques and represents the earliest form of the disease.

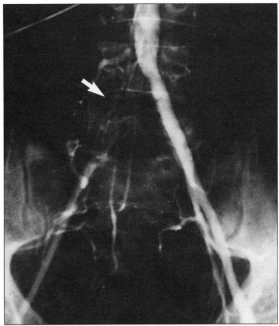

1.7 Peripheral arterial disease. This is most commonly symptomatic when affecting the carotid vessels and those of the lower limb. This angiogram shows an atheromatous block in the common iliac artery (arrow). This lesion produces the symptoms of claudication. The majority of patients with intermittent claudication stabilize or improve, but the disease progresses in a minority of patients (10–12%).

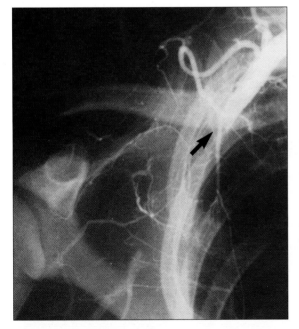

1.8 Peripheral arterial disease. PAD can also affect the upper limb. This angiogram demonstrates an atheromatous block in the axillary artery (arrow). Disease in this area produces arm claudication, often Raynaud's phenomenon, a diminished pulse on the affected side, and sometimes blanching on elevation of the limb.

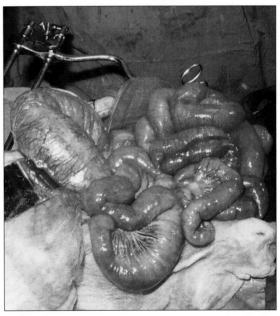

1.9 Mesenteric artery thrombosis. This can also result from atheromatous disease. In this perioperative slide, the pale and slightly discoloured bowel can be clearly seen.

VASOSPASM

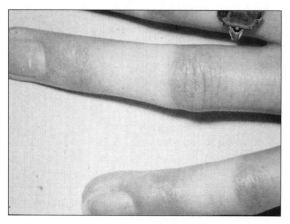

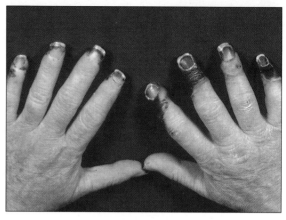

1.10 Raynaud's phenomenon. This is the commonest form of vasospasm, occurring in between 10 and 20% of young women. In the majority of cases the condition is benign: Raynaud's disease. Spasm of the small vessels in the fingers leads to the blanching seen here.

1.11 Raynaud's syndrome. When Raynaud's phenomenon occurs with an associated disorder it is called Raynaud's syndrome and produces more severe symptoms than its benign counterpart, Raynaud's disease. It may result in digital gangrene as seen here.

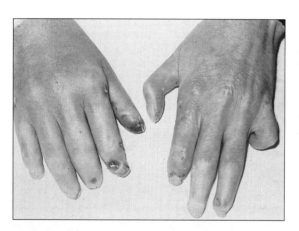

1.12 Severe Raynaud's syndrome. In severe disease there is usually a permanent obstructive element to the disorder in addition to the intermittent vasospasm. Some of the commonest groups of disorders associated with Raynaud's syndrome are the connective tissue diseases; in particular, 98% of patients with systemic sclerosis have Raynaud's syndrome. Intimal hyperplasia is the classical vascular lesion in systemic sclerosis and contributes to the severe ischaemia seen in this illustration.

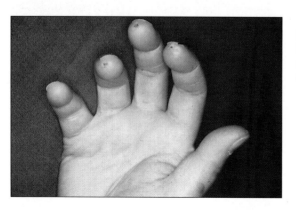

1.13 Digital pitting. The first sign of connective tissue disease in a patient who otherwise appears to have the benign form, Raynaud's disease, may be digital pitting. As shown here, these pits appear at the very tips of the digits and can develop into frank digital ulceration.

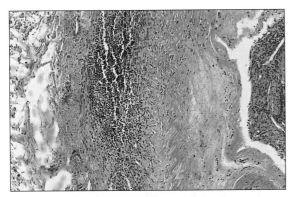

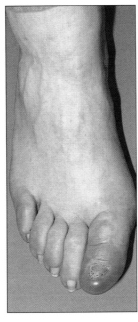

1.15 Buerger's disease (thromboangiitis obliterans). This may present with a cyanotic ischaemic digit, as seen here, in the presence of easily palpable peripheral pulses.

1.14 Buerger's disease (thromboangiitis obliterans). Another disorder commonly associated with Raynaud's syndrome is Buerger's disease, which occurs mainly in cigarette smokers with an onset at usually less than 45 years of age. The disease process has a predilection for the smaller blood vessels including those in both upper and lower limbs. Obliteration of the smaller blood vessels occurs with both smooth muscle cell proliferation and intraluminal thrombosis.

VASCULITIS

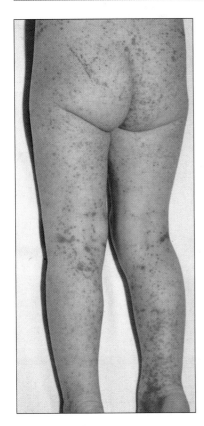

1.16 The vasculitides. These are characterized by inflammation of the blood vessel and are classified on the basis of involved vessel size and histology. An example of small vessel vasculitis is seen here in a patient suffering from Henoch–Schönlein purpura. A characteristic feature of small vessel vasculitis is a non-thrombo-cytopenic purpura caused by inflammation of the small cutaneous capillaries, particularly in the dependent parts of the body.

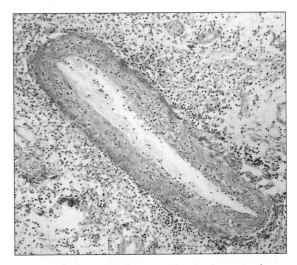

1.17 Pathology. Biopsy is central to the diagnosis of vasculitis and the changes seen on microscopy reflect a spectrum ranging from pure arteritis without granuloma formation to pure granulomatosis without vasculitis. Polyarteritis nodosa (PAN) and rheumatoid vasculitis are therefore at one end of the spectrum, while rheumatoid nodules and Wegener's granuloma are at the other. This illustration shows PAN in which muscular arteries throughout the body are involved. All layers of vessel wall are affected by fibrinoid necrosis and an inflammatory infiltrate of predominantly polymorphonuclear leucocytes.

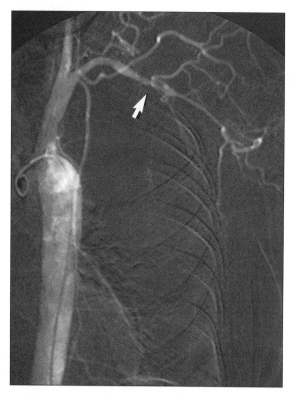

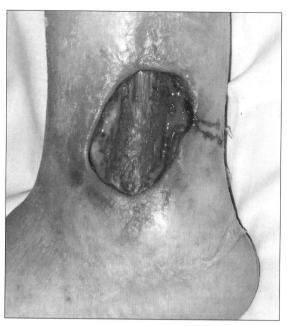

1.18 Takayasu's arteritis. This is a large vessel arteritis and is a rare disease that occurs predominantly in women. The arteritis involves the aortic arch and its branches. The inflammation results in stenosis, which may be demonstrated by arteriography, as shown here where there is narrowing in the left subclavian artery (arrow).

1.19 Skin manifestations of vasculitis. The commonest presentation of severe vasculitis is ulceration. Classically the lesion is 'punched out', as seen here, and often occurs in areas not usually associated with venous ulceration. As the development of vasculitic ulcers can be associated with internal organ involvement, and because their treatment involves the administration of potentially toxic drugs, a careful clinical history and examination must be combined with appropriate investigations. This patient has rheumatoid arthritis (RA) as detected by a positive RA latex test and has developed a vasculitic ulcer.

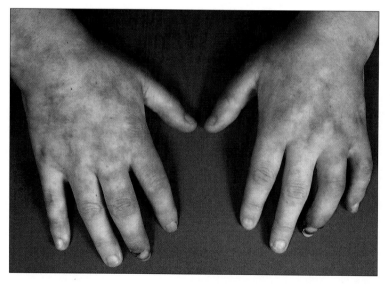

1.20 Aetiology. The skin can provide clues to the aetiology of leg ulceration. This illustration demonstrates livedo reticularis of the upper limb, which on biopsy will demonstrate the classical appearance of a vasculitis with polymorphonuclear infiltration.

2.

Risk Factors for Vascular Disease

The term 'risk factor' was first used in conjunction with the Framingham Heart Study, which was initiated in 1948 to evaluate factors associated with heart disease in a community 20 miles west of Boston, USA. Children of the original Framingham cohort were recruited in the early 1970s to participate in a similar study of risk factors, but this time vascular disease outwith the heart was also evaluated. These and other studies have provided us with evidence implicating certain behavioural and metabolic problems associated with the development of premature atherosclerotic peripheral vascular disease. The commonest cause of death is cardiovascular disease. Even those in the lowest risk category are still likely to die from cardiovascular disease, but they will develop the problem later in life. Risk factor detection allows therapy to be directed at those at risk of early-onset vascular disease. Not all risk factors can be modified, however, and these probably have most influence on the development of the disease.

Non-modifiable risk factors		Modifiable risk factors	
Major	**Minor**	**Major**	**Minor**
Increasing age	Soft water	Cigarette smoking	Obesity
Male sex	Hyperuricaemia	Hypertension	Stress
Positive family history	Type-A personality	Hyperlipidaemia	Lack of exercise
		Diabetes mellitus	? Abstinence from alcohol

2.1 Non-modifiable risk factors. Non-modifiable risk factors include male sex, older age and a strong family history of vascular disease. Men are more prone to the development of vascular disease, and women lose their presumed hormonal protection after the menopause, with the incidence of cardiovascular disease equalizing in those 70–80 years of age. Hormone replacement therapy has been shown (in early studies) to confer a continuation of this protection to postmenopausal women. It should be stressed that vascular disease in a menopausal female is not a contraindication to hormone replacement therapy. The risk of cardiovascular disease increases with increasing age and a strong family history of disease. However, this latter only holds true if the relative developed the disease before 60 years of age.

	European Atherosclerosis Society	US National Cholesterol Education Program
Acceptable cholesterol level	≤ 5.2 mmol/l	≤ 5.2 mmol/l
Dietary intervention	5.2–6.5 mmol/l	5.2–6.2 mmol/l
Drug therapy following trial of diet	6.5–7.8 mmol/l	6.2 mmol/l and above
Drug therapy probably after an inadequate dietary response	> 7.8 mmol/l	

2.2 Hyperlipidaemia. Hyperlipidaemia is associated with an increased risk of atherosclerosis. Risk can be reduced by decreasing cholesterol and triglyceride levels towards normal. Cholesterol-rich particles, particularly low density lipoproteins, are especially atherogenic. The World Health Organization recommendation for cholesterol is below 5.2 mmol/litre, although almost 50% of the population have levels of 6.5 mmol/litre or over. Consensus guidelines for the management of hypercholesterolaemia in Europe and the USA are shown here. Lipid levels may be disturbed for several weeks after severe stress such as an operative procedure or myocardial infarction and measurement should be delayed for some weeks afterwards.

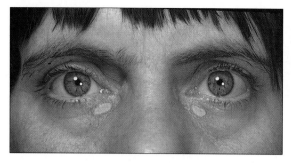

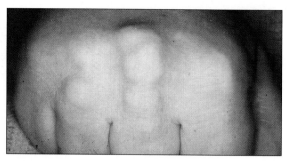

2.3 Cutaneous markers for hyperlipidaemia. These may be visible, for example the xanthelasma seen here. Xanthelasma is a small subcutaneous collection of lipid that gathers beneath the eye in a patient with hyperlipidaemia.

2.4 Xanthoma. This is a subcutaneous collection of lipid that tends to occur over a tendon or a point of prominence such as the elbow or knee. In this slide, tendon xanthomas can be clearly seen extending over the metacarpophalangeal joints.

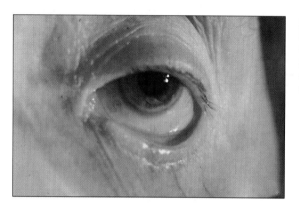

2.5 Corneal arcus. Another easily visible manifestation of hyperlipidaemia, if it occurs in the younger person, is corneal arcus. As senile arcus is very common in the elderly population, this marker of hyperlipidaemia is usually only clinically useful when detected in people under 70 years of age.

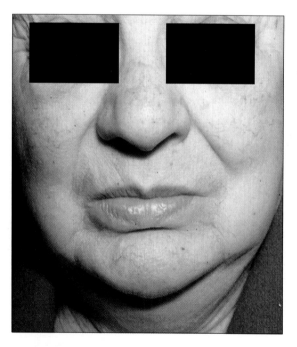

2.6 Secondary hyperlipidaemia. This may occur with hypothyroidism as illustrated in this picture. Note the puffy appearance of the face with obesity and coarsening of the features. Patients with severe hypothyroidism often have vascular disease and the introduction of thyroid hormone treatment must be gradual to avoid stressing a potentially impaired coronary circulation.

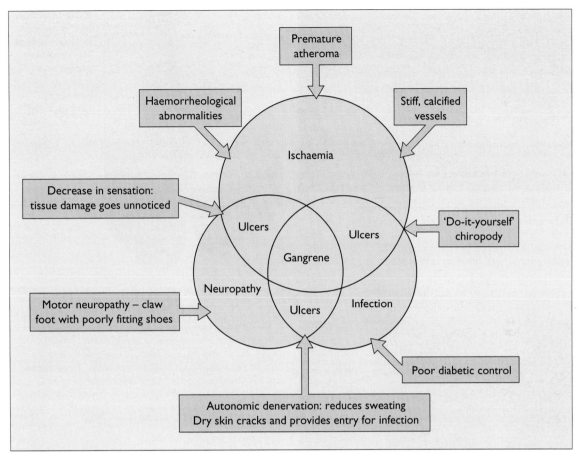

2.7 Diabetes mellitus. A major risk factor for the development of peripheral arterial disease is diabetes mellitus. A number of features contribute to this increased risk, including an abnormal lipid metabolism, increased oxidative stress and microvascular abnormalities. These combine to promote premature atherosclerosis and thus limb ischaemia. The diagram outlines the important abnormalities occurring in the diabetic foot. Between 50 and 70% of all amputations occur in diabetic patients, who have a 15 times greater risk of undergoing a major amputation than other vasculopaths. In the UK, 30% of all amputations that take place are in diabetics, and ultimately 5–15% of diabetic patients will experience some limb amputation process.

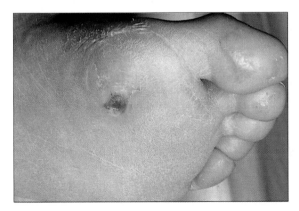

2.8 Ulceration. The commonest manifestation of diabetic foot problems is ulceration. Purely neuropathic ulcers occur at high pressure sites, as seen here, where a thinning of the skin of the toes is evident and ulceration has developed over a shoe pressure point.

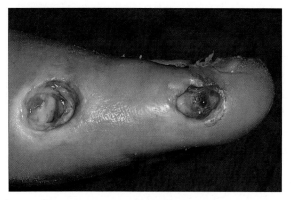

2.9 Neuropathy combined with pressure ischaemia. This commonly produces ulcers in the 'bunion' area. These ulcers in the diabetic can penetrate deeply down to the bone. Osteomyelitis in the diabetic foot is associated with a poor survival outcome for the limb.

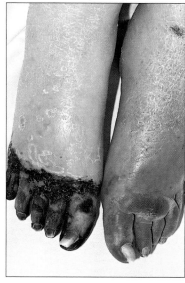

2.10 Infection in the neuro-ischaemic foot. This should be treated as a medical emergency because tissue destruction and gangrene can rapidly ensue.

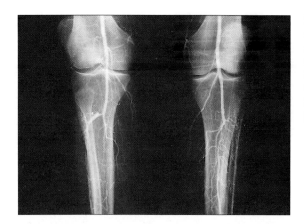

2.11 Angiographic investigation. The diabetic patient with peripheral arterial disease should always have an angiographic investigation because angioplasty and/or surgical reconstruction is frequently possible. Nevertheless, diabetic vascular disease has an unfortunate predilection for the three vessels below the knee and the 'run-off' patency of these and lower vessels is important with regard to vascular grafting and prognosis in the diabetic.

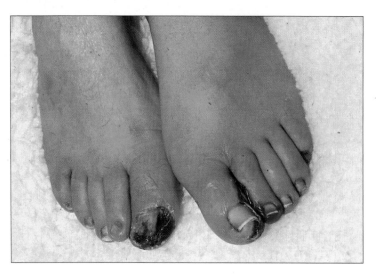

2.12 Distal disease. This 54-year-old patient has the typical ulceration and gangrene of the toes that is particularly seen in the diabetic with more pronounced distal disease.

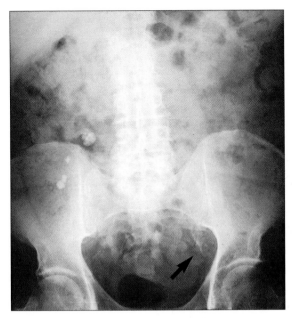

2.13 Ankle brachial blood pressure measurements. In the diabetic patient, these Doppler ultrasound measurements are notoriously unreliable as a guide to limb circulation because of the stiffening, and even calcification, of the vessels, as seen here. These vessels are non-compressible during the test and near-normal ankle brachial pressure ratios can be obtained if the calcification affects the distal vessels.

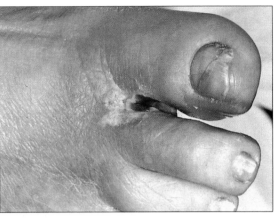

2.14 Treatment and investigation. Diabetic foot ulceration must be investigated and treated early. Ulcers, such as this one, seen here between the toes, must be aggressively treated if they are not to progress. Diabetic control must be good, and in addition to vascular tests, infection must be sought and the depth of the ulcer estimated from bone radiographs. Mechanisms that alleviate pressure on the area, such as bed rest or splinting, must be employed. Rocker shoes, which spread the pressure more evenly throughout the foot, can be of use for ulcers over the metatarsal heads or on the heels.

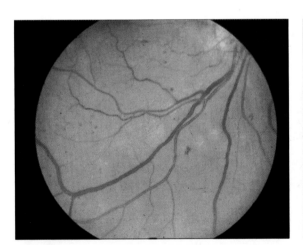

2.15 Background diabetic retinopathy. Diabetic vascular disease affects any vessel within the body. This includes the peripheral vessels in the limb, and carotid, coronary and retinal vessels. The initial changes seen on ophthalmoscopy show the classical dot and blot haemorrhages of background retinopathy.

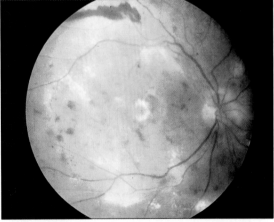

2.16 Exudative diabetic retinopathy. This is commonly found in type II non-insulin dependent diabetics. As such diabetic patients often have peripheral arterial disease of the lower limb, these fundoscopic findings are common in hospital vascular wards. This slide shows the dot and blot haemorrhages of background retinopathy, and also exudates, which result from the positioning and then death of lipid foam-filled macrophages in the retina. Appropriate modification of an abnormal lipid profile is important in the diabetic patient.

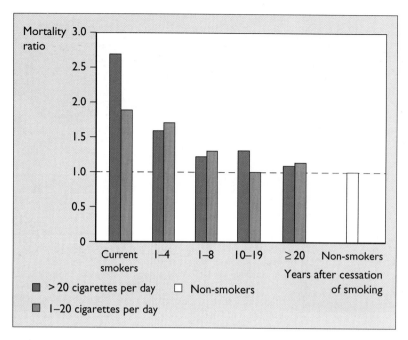

2.17 Smoking. The most important modifiable risk factor for peripheral arterial disease is probably smoking, especially of cigarettes, but also pipes and cigars if smoke is inhaled. Smoking not only contributes to the development and progression of this disease, but also to the failure of vascular grafts. The difficulty encountered by patients trying to give up smoking should not be underemphasized. Nevertheless, the successful cessation of smoking does have distinct health benefits, as can be seen in this figure.

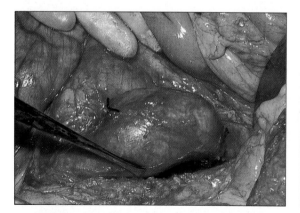

2.18 Nicotine. This is a highly addictive drug and patients should receive support in order to achieve a non-smoking status, which may include primary care counselling and/or nicotine patches. (Reproduced with the permission of Zyma Healthcare, Surrey, UK.)

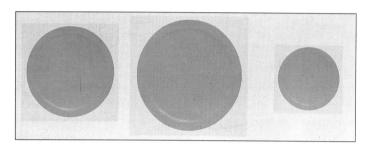

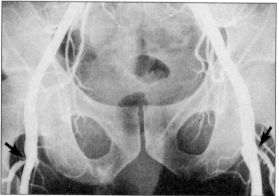

2.19 Hypertension. This is a well-recognized risk factor for coronary and carotid vascular disease, but the evidence for its role in peripheral arterial disease is less convincing, though the link between hypertension and the development of an aortic aneurysm is not in doubt. This aortic aneurysm was causing abdominal discomfort in an 82-year-old patient. Because the risk of rupture increases with the size of the aneurysm and the presence of pain, it was resected.

2.20 Increased vascular resistance. When combined with increased shear stresses produced by a high blood pressure, increased vascular resistance may also contribute to peripheral arterial disease in the lower limb, particularly so at the bifurcation of vessels. Stenoses of the origins of both profunda femoris arteries are seen in this film. It is important to detect this because if the superficial femoral artery is blocked, limb survival depends on the profunda flow.

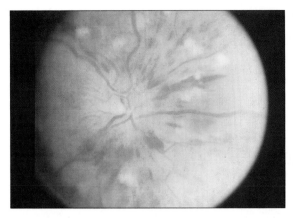

2.21 Hypertensive retinopathy. The first manifestation of hypertensive retinopathy is a silver-wiring appearance of the retinal vessels. This is followed by arteriovenous nipping and the later development of flame-shaped haemorrhages reflecting vessel rupture, and soft exudates reflecting retinal oedema. This illustration shows the appearances of the retina in a hypertensive crisis in which there is papilloedema and flame-shaped haemorrhages.

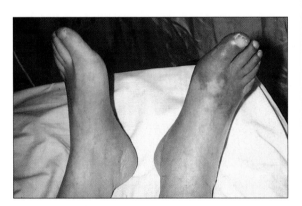

2.22 Critical limb ischaemia (CLI). This is a situation in which care must be taken when treating high blood pressure because in the acute early phase of CLI, an elevated pressure helps maintain perfusion of the affected limb. Nevertheless, continued hypertension will increase the incidence of cardiovascular complications such as stroke. Antihypertensive treatment could be deferred for a few weeks in the hospitalized patient with CLI whose systolic blood pressure is 180 mmHg or lower, and whose diastolic blood pressure is 100 mmHg or lower. If treatment is required, drugs with a vasodilatory effect are recommended, and nonselective beta-blockers should be avoided. Hypotensive shock has produced distal gangrene in this patient, but less severe 'hypotensive' episodes, even within the so-called normal range, may result in limb loss in CLI.

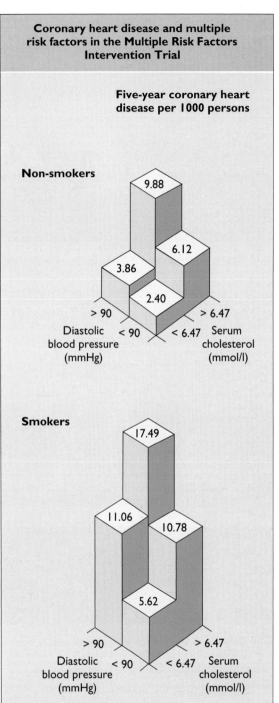

2.23 Combinations of risk factors. Risk factors tend to be synergistic. In the coronary circulation the risk of disease is trebled by the addition of cigarette smoking to a hypercholesterolaemic subject. The mechanisms whereby risk is multiplied rather than added probably include the cigarette smoke-induced oxidation of lipoproteins. (Reproduced with the permission of Merck, Sharp & Dohme Ltd.)

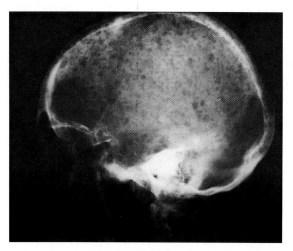

2.24 Hyperviscosity syndromes. These syndromes can also contribute to the development of poor circulatory flow and thrombosis. Multiple myeloma, in which there is neoplastic proliferation of plasma cells, is a well-recognized hyperviscosity syndrome that can present with unexplained peripheral arterial thrombotic disease. This radiograph of a skull shows the classical pepperpot lesions produced by multiple myeloma deposits in the bones.

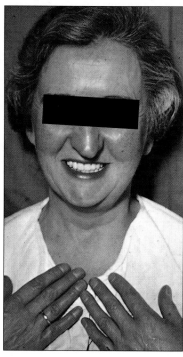

2.25 Polycyth-aemia rubra vera. This is a neoplastic proliferation of the red blood cells, and in this primary form there is also an increase in the platelet and white cell count. Facial plethora, as is seen here, is often a cardinal feature. Secondary polycythaemia is common in patients with peripheral arterial disease secondary to their smoking habit.

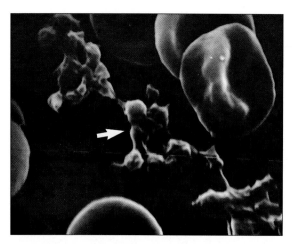

2.26 Other risk factors for vascular disease. These include haemorrheological abnormalities such as increased platelet aggregation, as seen here viewed by electron microscopy.

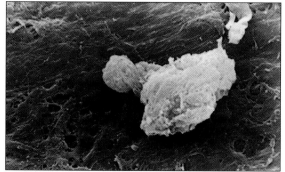

2.27 White blood cell activation. This has also been implicated in both atherogenesis and acute thrombosis, both of which are important in vascular disease. This activated white cell viewed by electron microscopy was taken from a patient with critical limb ischaemia. Other coagulation abnormalities have also been linked to the development of vascular disease, including abnormalities of blood clotting factors such as fibrinogen and factor VII.

3.

Examination of the Vascular Tree

Following a detailed history, a good and structured examination is the key to diagnosis in arterial and venous disease. This comprises inspection, palpation and auscultation, and occasionally percussion, as well as certain specific bedside tests. Inspection is a key area in the examination of the vascular system and the diagnosis will often be made following a good initial inspection alone.

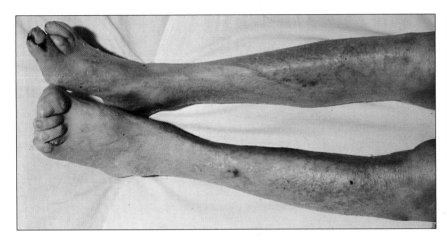

3.1 Hair loss. This finding is common in older patients, and although regularly found in arterial insufficiency and thus often taught to medical students as a classic sign of lower limb ischaemia, it is not necessarily pathogno-monic of this condition. Socks that are too tight can also contribute to hair loss.

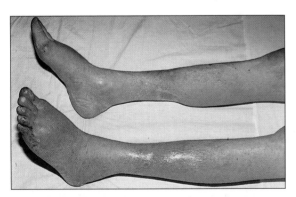

3.2 Leg swelling. Unilateral leg swelling is generally associated with venous obstruction or insufficiency, lymphatic disease or inflammation. It is not normally found in arterial disease, but chronic dependency (as in rest pain) may lead to marked dependent oedema. This slide shows the severe swelling that may occur with chronic rest pain. The patient slept upright every night, resulting in oedema of both legs, more marked in the left (ischaemic) foot.

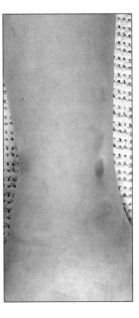

3.3 Pitting oedema. Many patients with peripheral vascular disease have associated cardiac decompensation, which may manifest as dyspnoea and ankle oedema, as seen here. It is important to reduce this form of oedema to a minimum in patients with critical ischaemia because significant oedema will further compromise the ischaemic lower limb.

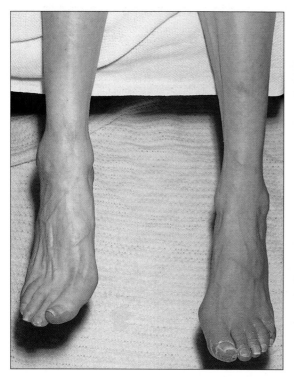

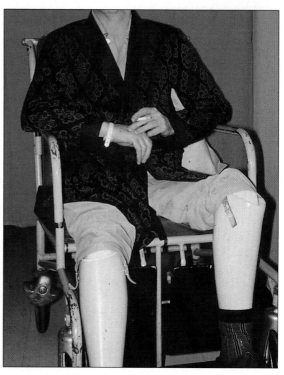

3.4 Colour changes. Many venous and arterial problems lead to alterations in skin colour and these are often best seen by comparing one limb with the other. In this case severe limb ischaemia is present in the left foot with a paradoxical rubor because of dependency. This redness is, however, classically cold and will disappear on elevation.

3.5 Loss of limbs/digits. The obvious should never be overlooked! Failure to examine the limbs properly may lead to considerable embarrassment later, as in this man who has had bilateral below knee amputations, but is otherwise very mobile and still smoking!

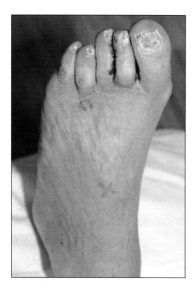

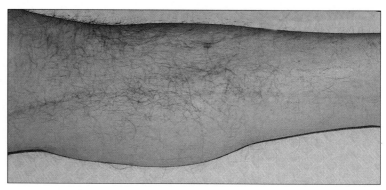

3.6 Ulceration. It is very important to look between the toes for trophic lesions, which may otherwise go unrecognized, especially in diabetic patients, as seen here.

3.7 Scars. Many vascular patients have had previous reconstructive operations and the scars from these operations should be noted. Occasionally, these can be misleading, as in this patient who has claudication, but who actually had his saphenous vein harvested for a coronary artery bypass.

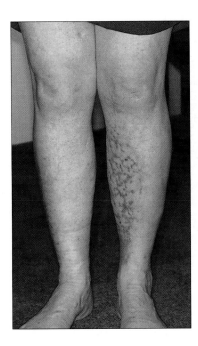

3.8 Erythema ab igne. This is a sign commonly seen in patients who sit too close to a fire, with resulting haemolysis of red cells and pigmentation in the classical reticular form. The astute clinician may be able to deduce on which side of the fire the patient prefers to sit!

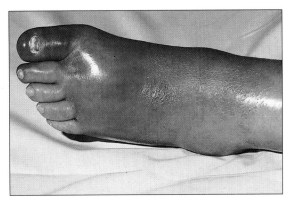

3.9 Cellulitis. Many patients present with a minor infection of the toe, which because of inadequate blood flow spreads to the whole foot and ultimately the leg. In diabetic patients this may become an emergency situation in which many organisms (both aerobic and anaerobic) are involved in the infective process. Urgent control of such infection with aggressive antibiotic therapy and adequate debridement or amputation may be necessary to save a limb and/or life.

PULSES

Pulses are often difficult to examine well and either not documented at all or not graded appropriately. The following simple system is recommended for grading all peripheral pulses.

- 0, absent.
- +, present, but diminished.
- ++, present and normal.
- +++, aneurysmal.

In general pulses should be examined in a warm environment and the examiner's hands should be warm, but not overly so. If the hands are too warm, it is easy to palpate one's own pulse against a solid structure such as the patient's metatarsal and mistake it for the patient's pulse.

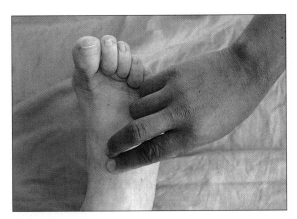

3.10 The dorsalis pedis pulse. This pulse is felt just lateral to the extensor hallucis longus tendon, and just below the ankle joint in the same line as the anterior tibial pulse.

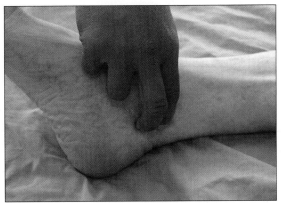

3.11 The posterior tibial pulse. Usually felt in the groove about 1 cm behind the medial malleolus, this pulse can be surprisingly difficult to feel in some patients even when there is no arterial disease.

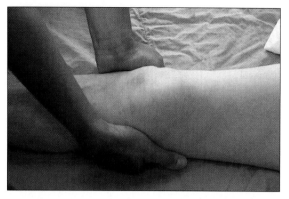

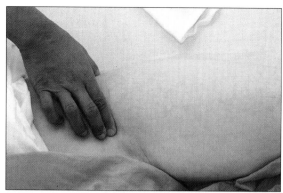

3.12 The popliteal pulse. This is most easily felt with the knee flexed either against the tibial plateau (as shown) or with the patient supine and by direct pressure against the femur. Even if present it is often very difficult to feel this pulse in the obese and heavily muscled patient.

3.13 The femoral pulse. This pulse is felt at the mid-inguinal point and should be compared in volume with that on the other side. If it is diminished, a 'thrill' may sometimes be felt and a bruit heard. This would suggest a proximal arterial narrowing.

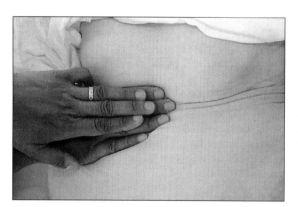

3.14 The aorta. An abdominal examination should always be performed in patients with a history of claudication, in whom there is a one in ten chance of finding an aortic aneurysm; however, many patients will be too obese for a definitive diagnosis to be made on clinical examination alone. Auscultation should also be performed to listen for bruits, which may emanate from the diseased aorta or one of its major branches. It is usually not possible to be specific about which visceral branch is responsible for a bruit which is clinically audible.

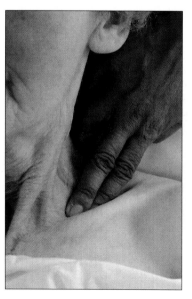

3.15 The subclavian artery. Despite its name, the subclavian artery is generally best felt just above the clavicle, as here. The axillary artery, which is its continuity can be felt inferior to the lateral half of the clavicle deep to pectoralis minor.

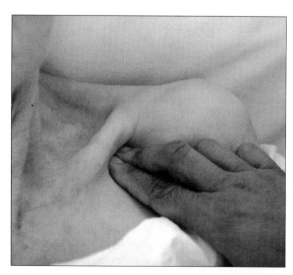

3.16 The axillary artery. This may be easily palpated in the axilla or below the distal third of the clavicle, as here.

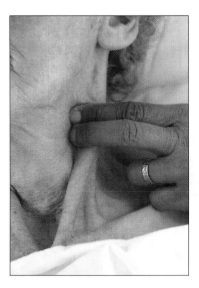

3.17 The carotid artery. This artery may be felt along the anterior border of sternomastoid. In thin individuals it is easily detected, but in the obese neck it can be surprisingly difficult to palpate.

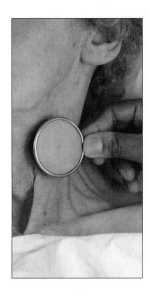

3.18 Auscultation of the carotid arteries. As depicted here, auscultation of the carotid arteries often elicits bruits in patients with vascular disease, but it may be difficult to determine whether the bruit comes from the common, internal or external carotid vessel. Most bruits probably arise from the external carotid and are therefore of limited clinical relevance beyond serving as a definite 'marker' of vascular disease.

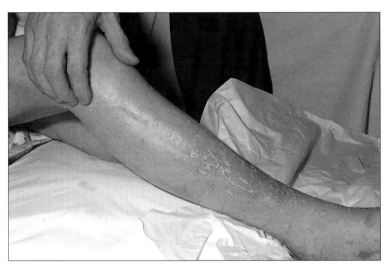

3.19 Superficial arterial grafts. These may also be easily palpated when present and should be carefully documented. Here, a long vein graft is palpable just beneath the skin surface as it winds its way down to the mid-peroneal artery.

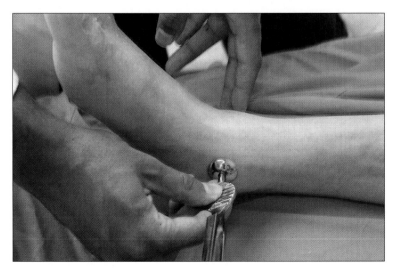

3.20 Loss of vibration sense. This is a valuable early finding in patients with peripheral vascular disease and diabetes mellitus. These patients have a particular risk of developing neurotrophic skin ulceration because of subsequent sensory neuropathy and therefore all 'at risk' patients should be appropriately tested. It should be remembered, however, that it is a common finding in general in patients aged 80 years or above.

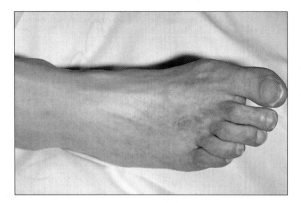

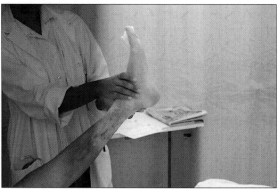

3.21 Prolonged venous guttering. After emptying the veins from the foot prolonged venous guttering is a cardinal sign of critical ischaemia. Here, the veins have not yet filled after 60 seconds of perfusion and the foot remains pale.

3.22 Buerger's test. Elevation of the leg in a patient with critical ischaemia results in the foot becoming bloodless. The angle of hip flexion at which this occurs and the subsequent length of time needed to restore perfusion (after letting the leg hang down again) provides a good index of the severity of arterial compromise.

4.

Investigation of the Vascular Tree

Vascular investigations play a very important role in the management of patients with peripheral vascular disease. In particular, the noninvasive vascular laboratory now provides a means of screening for disease, measuring severity and assessing results after intervention.

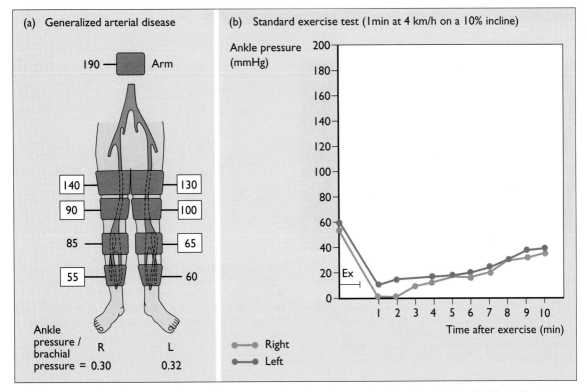

4.1 Doppler-derived segmental systolic pressures. With or without exercise testing, this is the main noninvasive investigation used in the detection of large vessel peripheral vascular disease. Cuffs are placed down the legs. On deflation the lowest systolic pressure at which flow is detected (using continuous wave Doppler ultrasound) is an indirect measurement of the arterial pressure in that vessel.

An index may be derived, which is called the A/B ratio (or ankle/arm index), by dividing the arm systolic pressure by the ankle pressure. This test may be further enhanced by exercising the patient. In normal subjects, exercise increases the systolic pressure in both the arm and leg; in the claudicant, the systolic pressure rises in the arm, but the ankle pressure falls, as demonstrated here. Ex = exercise.

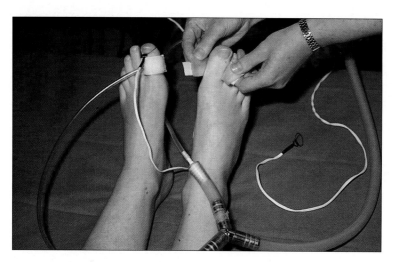

4.2 Toe pressure measurements.
These are very useful in the assessment of critical ischaemia where there is limb arterial wall stiffening, as occurs commonly in diabetic patients. The digital arteries are relatively spared and indirect pressure measurement here is therefore more meaningful. Detection of blood flow is usually by means of an infrared photodetector or by a strain gauge technique.

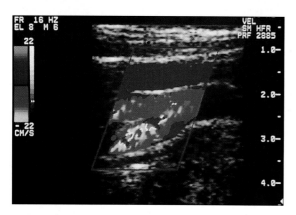

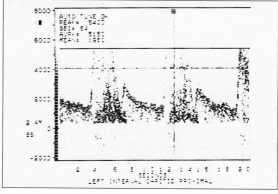

4.3 Duplex scanning. This provides both flow dynamics and an image of the vessel under investigation. It combines pulsed Doppler waveform analysis with B-mode Doppler images of the vessel in such a way that it is possible to focus the pulsed wave Doppler at exactly the right point and angle in the vessel. With colour-coded velocities, it provides great detail on flow dynamics and can be used to indirectly measure actual flow.

4.4 Waveform analysis is perhaps best used in the extracranial carotid arteries, as shown here, with the image (**4.3**) and the waveform analysis demonstrating a tight internal carotid lesion, but is increasingly used in the peripheral arterial tree to detect stenoses and occlusions as well as in arterial graft surveillance.

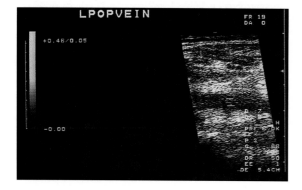

4.5 Venous duplex examination. This is now accepted as the first-line investigation for detecting significant lower and upper limb deep vein thrombosis (DVT). It is noninvasive, quick, repeatable and cheap. Although the test suffers from a degree of operator dependence, it is able to detect most clinically relevant DVTs above the knee. It is poor at detecting calf vein thrombosis.

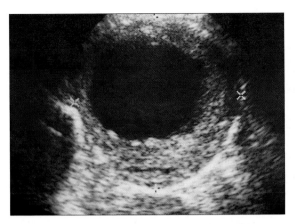

4.6 B-mode ultrasound. This is commonly used to detect aneurysms. The excellent spatial resolution now available with modern machines makes this the main method for screening for aortic aneurysm because it gives an accurate indication of luminal and total vessel diameter.

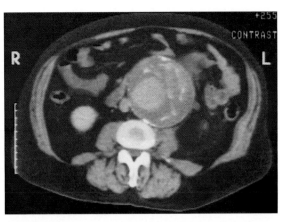

4.7 Computed tomography (CT) scanning. This can be used in the assessment of doubtful aneurysms or where there is a suspicion of suprarenal involvement of the aneurysm. In this case, the aneurysm is confined to the infrarenal aorta.

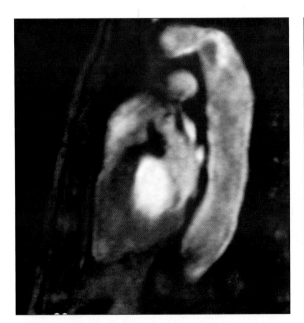

4.8 Magnetic resonance imaging (MRI). These techniques have developed rapidly and are now becoming available to most regional vascular centres. Unfortunately the image quality of most machines is not yet adequate to replace angiography for the routine investigation of the arterial tree. MRI costs suggest that ultrasound imaging will remain the main methodology for the initial screening of vessels in the immediate future.

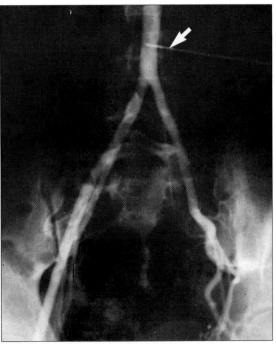

4.9 Translumbar angiogram. This was the original method of obtaining radiographic images. Here, a percutaneous needle is placed in the aorta and dye injected. This required a general anaesthetic and an inpatient hospital stay. The percutaneous needle is indicated (arrow).

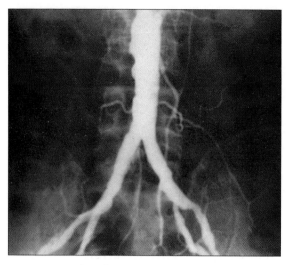

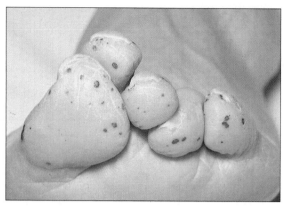

4.11 Embolization after arteriography.
Complications during and following angiography occur in 1–4% of cases. They are usually mild and limited to bruising around the site of catheter insertion. In this case, small microemboli have been dislodged by the placement of the catheter resulting in these purpuric-type lesions in the toes; healing was uneventful.

4.10 Conventional angiograms. These are now routinely performed using a Seldinger technique where a guide wire is inserted into the femoral artery and a catheter railroaded over this up to the aorta. Transaortic arteriograms are now almost never indicated and with the small size of catheters used currently, day-case and outpatient angiography is easily and safely performed with only a small risk of bleeding (*see* **6.53**).

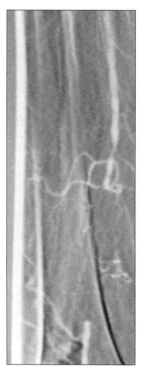

4.12 Intra-arterial digital subtraction angiogram (i.a. DSA). This uses a computerized method and a small amount of contrast material and 'subtracts' a pre-contrast image from the image with contrast, therefore, in theory, leaving only an image of contrast material. As a result only very small catheters and a low volume of contrast material are needed. However, the image is not as clear as that of a standard angiogram.

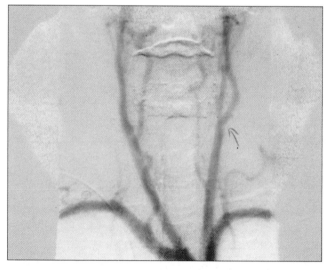

4.13 Intravenous digital subtraction angiography (i.v. DSA). A catheter is placed in the superior vena cava and a large bolus of contrast injected. Using the same techniques as for intra-arterial DSA, reasonable images of the proximal arterial system can be obtained. This method is very useful in cases of aortoiliac occlusion, but in general, does not allow imaging of the distal leg arteries.

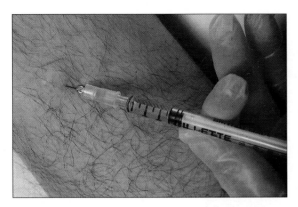

4.14 Skin blood flow measurements. Skin blood flow measurements can be performed using an intradermal injection technique of an isotope such as iodine-125 iodoantipyrine. After injection of this radioisotope into the dermis of the skin, the resultant washout can be measured using a sodium iodine crystal and amplifier and the clearance measured using a logged curve such as that shown here. Generally speaking, this technique is reserved for amputation level selection or research purposes, and may become further limited with the recent radioisotope control legislation.

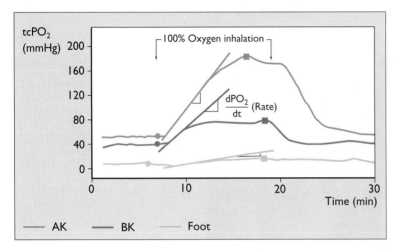

4.15 Transcutaneous oxygen measurements (tcPO$_2$). These measurements, which were originally designed to reflect intra-arterial oxygen tension in the neonate, have been commonly applied to the assessment of skin viability in the ischaemic limb. This slide shows measurements obtained at the above-knee, below-knee and foot levels, and the result of giving the patient 100% oxygen. It can be seen that there is a very poor response in the foot and indeed this patient had a critically ischaemic limb.

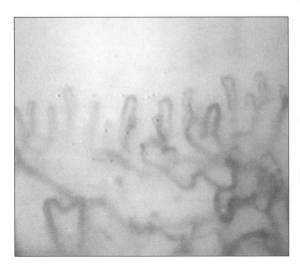

4.16 Capillary microscopy. This technique is used to assess the morphology and flow in the capillary bed. It is most useful in the nailfold beds where assessment is easy. This picture shows a normal nailfold pattern seen at the finger nailfold.

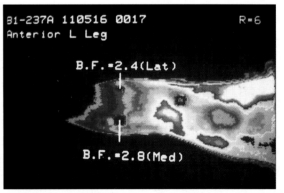

4.17 Infrared thermography. This infrared thermogram of a critically ischaemic limb before amputation shows a steep thermal gradient at a level approximately 15 cm distal to the tibial tuberosity. Skin blood measurements have been superimposed on the medial and lateral aspects of the leg and are measured in ml/100 g of tissue/min. Thermography can usefully predict amputation level and can demonstrate the viability of skin flaps in difficult below-knee amputations.

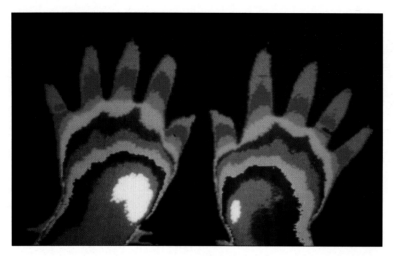

4.18 Thermography in Raynaud's phenomenon.
Thermography can be usefully employed to measure the rewarming time following cold challenge. This illustration shows cold blue fingers, the tips of which are so cold that they blend into the background, producing the so-called thermographic amputation picture. Moving more proximally the hand and wrist and lower arm can be seen to be increasingly warm.

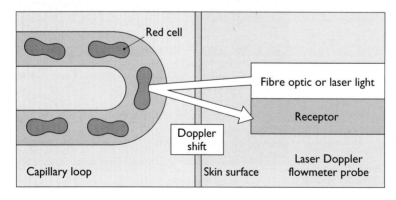

4.19 Thermography in Raynaud's phenomenon.
Thermography can also be helpful in predicting progression to connective tissue disease. Bilateral symmetrical disease, as seen in **4.18**, is usually linked to benign primary Raynaud's disease. In contrast, unilateral Raynaud's phenomenon, affecting the left hand as seen here, tends to be found in patients who are destined to develop a connective tissue disease such as systemic sclerosis.

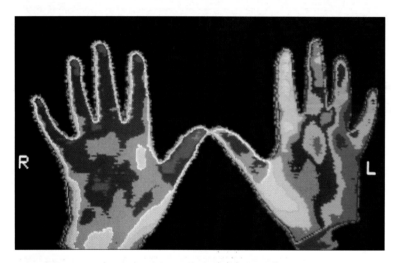

4.20 Laser Doppler flowmetry (LDF).
The principle underlying LDF is the same as in ultrasound and measures flow in vessels. In this technique, a narrow beam of monochromatic light is generated by a low-power laser and carried by an optical fibre to the skin. Light hitting moving blood cells will undergo a slight Doppler shift, but light hitting static structures will be unchanged.

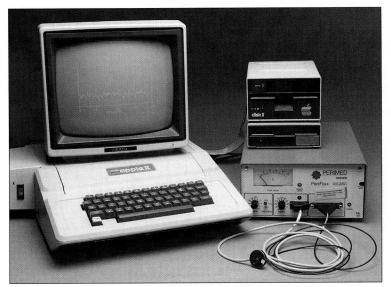

4.21 Laser Doppler flowmetry.
The magnitude and frequency distribution of the Doppler shift are directly related to the numbers and velocities of blood cells; therefore, a cell motion-correlated signal, the red blood cell flux, is obtained. An output signal in volts is generated, which is linearly related to the red blood cell flux. This output signal can be captured on a visual display unit, as shown here, or on a chart recorder.

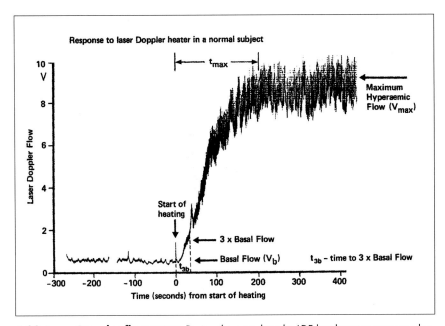

4.22 Laser Doppler flowmetry. During the past decade, LDF has become very popular as a means of evaluating skin microcirculation. Nevertheless, certain considerations must be given to the interpretation of the output signals. Biological zero values should be subtracted from the values recorded and the instrument should only be used in a temperature-controlled environment. A skin heater can be attached to the probe to allow standardized heating of the skin surrounding the area being studied. Therefore, in addition to providing a measurement of basal blood flow, the technique also allows an estimation of vasodilatation in response to heat. Both the speed of the vasodilator response and the extent of the response can be measured.

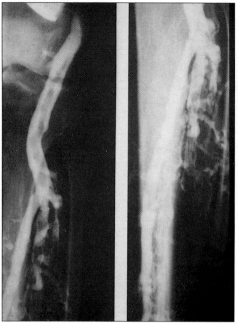

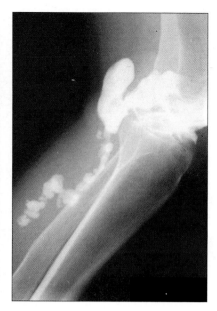

4.24 Arthrogram. One of the differential diagnoses of a deep vein thrombosis is a ruptured Baker's cyst presenting as a painful swollen calf. This arthrogram clearly demonstrates the cyst behind the knee, with contrast tracking down into the calf showing rupture of the cyst. Ultrasonic duplex scanning is also useful in detecting these cysts, though less useful if the cyst has ruptured and emptied.

4.23 Venogram. Venography has been the gold standard for the detection of abnormalities in the venous system, particularly in the lower leg. This picture shows the presence of thrombus in the popliteal and tibial veins. Note the clot lying along the middle of the vein depicted as a filling defect.

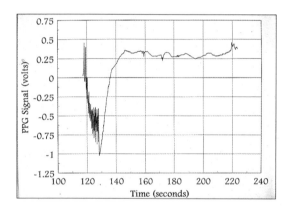

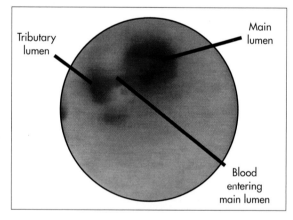

4.25 Venous photoplethysmography. A functional assessment of the venous system may be obtained using a noninvasive technique to measure venous refilling. Here, the patient has a photoplethysmographic probe placed on the lower leg when standing upright. He is then asked to stand up and down on his toes for about 20 cycles. This results in a fall in venous pressure and a drop in voltage detected by the system. He then stands still and the rate of refilling may be assessed. Here, there is very prompt refilling (less than 8 s), suggesting valvular incompetence. Placing appropriate venous tourniquets allows the method to discriminate between deep and superficial venous incompetence.

4.26 Angioscopy. This technique has recently become widely available to the vascular clinician although its exact role has yet to be clearly defined. Here, it is being used to examine a saphenous vein at the time of preparation during a distal *in situ* bypass. A tributary is clearly seen coming in from the left with blood entering the main stream. Using this system it is possible, though tricky, to limit the extent of exposure of the vein when doing a distal bypass in the hope of reducing wound problems.

5.

Acute Ischaemia

The causes of acute ischaemia of the limb are summarized in **5.1**. Nowadays, acute ischaemia is most commonly seen in the older population and the diagnosis is unfortunately often initially overlooked, especially in old people's homes and geriatric wards, and even in acute medical and surgical wards.

Causes of acute ischaemia
Embolism
Thrombosis
Acute dissection
Trauma
Compression
Intra-arterial injections
Cold injury
Severe vasospasm

5.1 Causes of acute ischaemia.

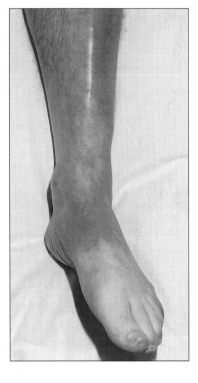

5.2 Acute ischaemia of the leg. The foot is white and demonstrates the classical 'six Ps': pulseless, painful, pale, paraesthesia, paralysis and perishing cold. It has not yet reached the stage of 'fixed mottling' and is therefore potentially salvageable with either thrombolysis or surgery. Early intervention is needed with angiography and surgery or thrombolysis.

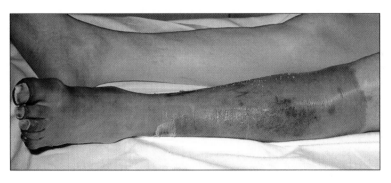

5.3 Acute ischaemia. In this case, the late changes of fixed mottling and irreversible ischaemia have developed. Revascularization at this stage is not only futile, but may be fatal, with the release of endotoxins and free radicals contributing to renal failure and multisystemic failure. Primary amputation was required.

EMBOLISM

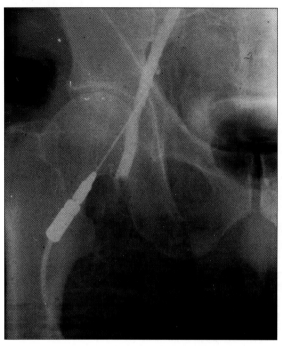

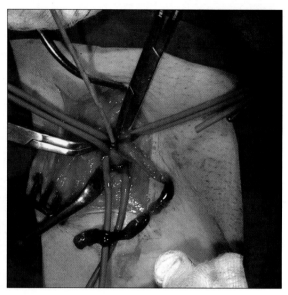

5.4 Embolus in the right femoral artery. The arteriogram shows an embolus, recognized by the crescenteric appearance at the lower part of the contrast material, in the right common femoral artery. With an acute embolus, there is usually no history of claudication and there is usually an underlying potential primary source such as a recent myocardial infarct, atrial fibrillation or proximal aneurysm.

5.5 Embolus in the right femoral artery. An embolus is being removed from the right femoral artery using a Fogarty catheter. In a good embolectomy, the catheter slips past the clot easily and most of the clot can be removed. However, some clot will inevitably remain and 'on-table' thrombolysis may be beneficial by instilling tissue plasminogen activator down the vessel. Where embolectomy is difficult or impossible, there is almost certainly underlying atherosclerotic disease and the patient will require femoropopliteal or distal bypass grafting. Therefore embolectomy should generally only be carried out by a surgeon capable of going on to reconstruction if necessary.

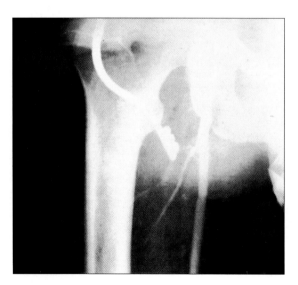

5.6 Embolus in the right femoral artery. The embolus has been removed and a completion angiogram obtained, which now demonstrates good flow down the superficial femoral artery. Views should also be taken of the popliteal trifurcation to ensure that at least one tibial vessel is adequately perfused. Most patients will require postoperative anticoagulation.

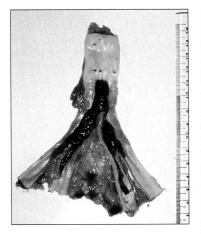

5.7 Saddle embolus. An embolus lodging at the aortic bifurcation is a most serious event that will usually result in death unless promptly dealt with by bilateral femoral embolectomy. This patient had a sudden onset of pain in both legs with a subsequent loss of power in the legs and lower abdominal wall mottling. The diagnosis was made too late to save the patient.

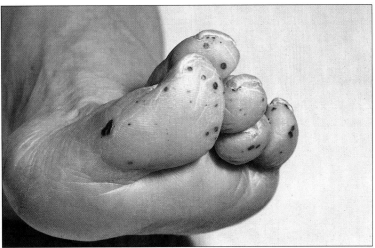

5.8 Microemboli in toes. Showers of small emboli may lead to the effect seen here where little areas of pinpoint necrosis occur. The feet are otherwise warm, often with palpable pedal pulses.

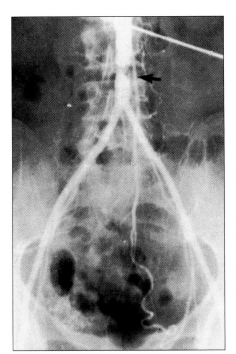

5.9 Aortic stenosis. This is an obvious source of embolization, which in the past would have required major surgery. Aortic balloon angioplasty with or without stenting is the optimal treatment here.

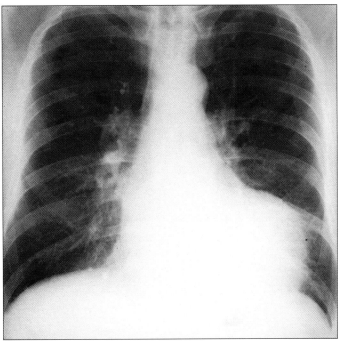

5.10 Aneurysm of the left ventricle. A rare source of arterial embolism is seen here in which the embolism has arisen some months after a myocardial infarct. Remember, however, that acute myocardial infarction itself is a common cause of embolization arising from endocardial mural thrombus.

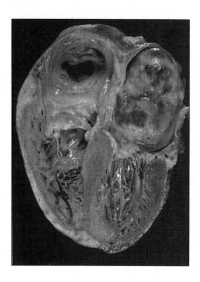

5.11 Myxoma of left atrium. Another rare cause of arterial embolization is seen here. This atrial tumour can be seen almost completely filling the left atrium. Histopathology showed it to be a myxoma. Death was caused by obstruction of the mitral valve and cardiac arrest.

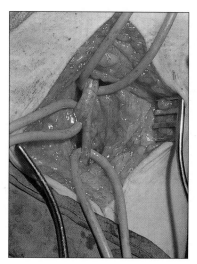

5.12 Atrial myxoma embolus. Though classically taught as one of the causes of arterial embolus, atrial myxoma embolus is very rarely seen. The unusual appearance of odd material extruding from the aortic arteriotomy is seen here framed by the rubber sling.

ACUTE THROMBOSIS

Acute thrombosis is rarely seen without an underlying precipitating factor. In most cases, there is a pre-existing atherosclerotic lesion, although other factors such as cardiac failure or cold may be the main exacerbating features.

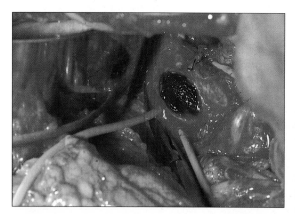

5.13 Acute spontaneous aortic thrombosis. This catastrophic event is occasionally seen and often diagnosed late. The patient may complain of sudden severe pain in the lower abdomen and legs with coldness and perhaps paralysis of the lower limbs. Without emergency intervention, death is almost certain if there has been no previous occlusive aortoiliac disease (and therefore no collaterals). In spontaneous cases that survive, a possible underlying collagen vascular disease may be present and should be looked for.

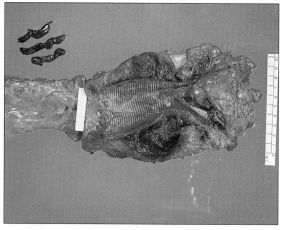

5.14 Acute aortic graft thrombosis. Following the repair of a ruptured aortic aneurysm with a bifurcation graft, this patient developed an acutely ischaemic right leg. Exploration of the femoral artery revealed thrombus, which probably developed at the time of cross-clamping without heparin. The patient subsequently died of renal failure. It is important to remember that disruption of arterial flow is a major cause of intravascular thrombosis.

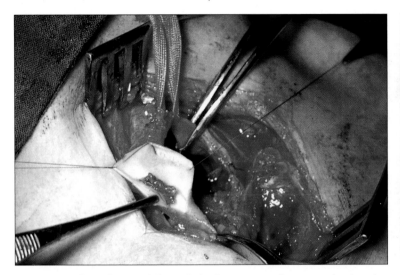

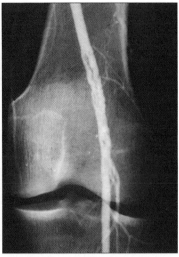

5.15 Acute thrombosis of the subclavian artery. This patient developed an acutely ischaemic arm secondary to subclavian artery thrombosis. At exploration the clot was easily removed and was noted to be secondary to a stenosis caused by a cervical rib. In such cases it is vital to perform an adequate thoracic outlet decompression with excision of the cervical rib and possibly of the first rib too.

5.16 Acute popliteal artery thrombosis. This arteriogram shows clot in the popliteal artery. This may be either embolus or thrombus. The ideal treatment here is to perform thrombolysis with tissue plasminogen activator (tPA) or streptokinase to clear the clot, and then to repeat the angiograms looking for the underlying cause.

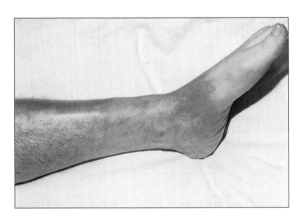

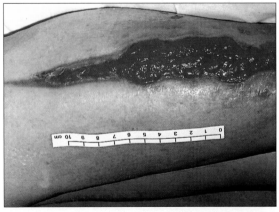

5.17 Acute femoral thrombosis. This leg shows the classical 'six Ps'. Although thrombolysis may be an option in many cases, the presence of such severe ischaemia necessitates emergency surgery with embolectomy and 'on-table' angiography if the limb is to be saved. 'On-table' thrombolysis is often beneficial for more peripheral embolization down the calf.

5.18 Fasciotomy. If limb ischaemia is very severe, a lower limb fasciotomy is often required to prevent secondary muscle ischaemia due to swelling of the muscles and subsequent compartment syndrome. If in doubt, it is better to perform fasciotomies because to do one 'later' is often 'too late'.

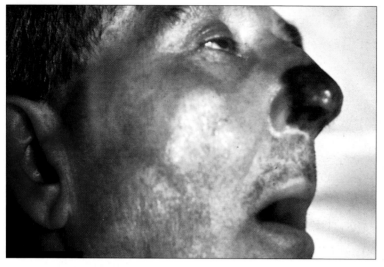

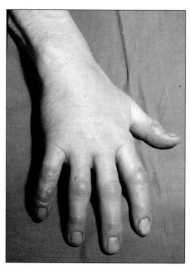

5.19 End-stage cardiac failure. In this patient, cardiac failure secondary to myocardial infarction has led to severe peripheral circulatory failure with early gangrene of the nose. More usually the toes and fingers would be involved in such a severe case.

5.20 Cold-induced arterial injury. This is less commonly seen now. This patient has early 'frostbite' of the fingers. Note the swelling and blisters.

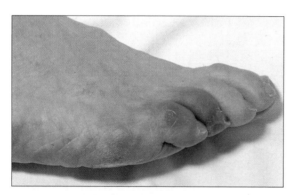

5.21 Cold-induced arterial injury involving the right foot. This patient was found outside in the snow; foot pulses were present. Treatment with heparin and prostacyclin or its synthetic analogues is likely to improve the circulation considerably.

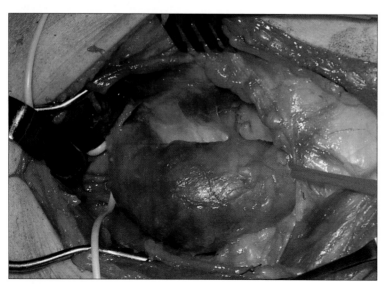

5.22 Popliteal aneurysm thrombosis. Although embolization of thrombus from these aneurysms is more common, an acute thrombosis of the aneurysm may occur. This can be a fairly devastating event, with an exacerbation of the clinical situation by microemboli. Emergency surgery with popliteal bypass and 'on-table' thrombolysis of the distal circulation offers the best chance of limb salvage, but despite this, major amputation may be required if gangrene has set in.

TRAUMA

Knife and gunshot wounds are occurring with increasing frequency in urban communities, and occasionally involve a major vessel with resultant acute ischaemia. The presence of a pulse detected by Doppler ultrasound is insufficient evidence of arterial patency in these cases and where any doubt exists emergency arteriography should be performed

without delay. Failure to do so may result in a failure to rescue a marginally viable limb.

Acute venous thrombosis may be just as serious as primary arterial occlusion. In severe cases, arterial ischaemia will occur as a secondary phenomenon to the obstructed blood flow.

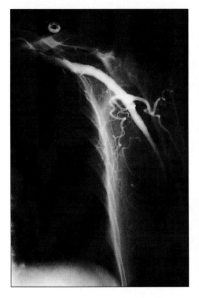

5.23 Emergency arteriogram.
This was carried out in a young man who sustained a compression injury to the upper arm without a skin laceration after being caught in a tractor power take-off mechanism. The arm was cold and pale and the arteriogram suggested 'spasm' of the brachial artery with occlusion.

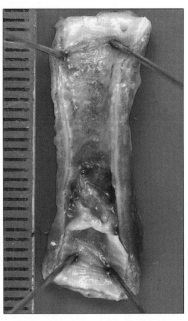

5.24 Intimal injury. At operation, an intimal transection and consequent flap was found with secondary thrombosis. Resection of the lesion and end-to-end anastomosis after mobilizing the artery was possible with an excellent end-result.

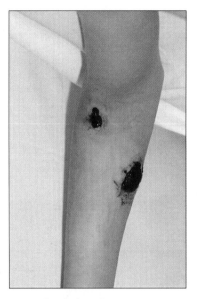

5.25 Blood clot. This patient was injured by broken plate glass, a piece of which had penetrated his forearm. Exploration of the wound in casualty failed to detect an arterial injury. Profuse recurrent bleeding resulted in contracture of the elbow and the patient was taken to theatre for formal exploration.

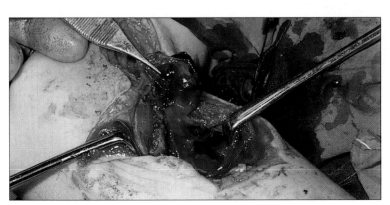

5.26 False traumatic aneurysm.
At operation, a traumatic aneurysm of a large muscular branch of the ulnar artery supplying the forearm muscles was found. This had bled under the deep fascia and caused an early compression problem at the elbow. Simple ligation and debridement was all that was required.

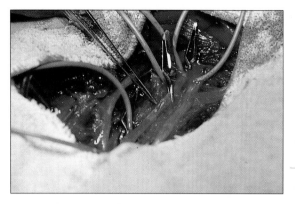

5.27 Stab injury to the axillary artery. Knife injuries are an increasing problem in urban society. In this case the axillary artery was transfixed, but is relatively accessible. It is far more difficult to gain quick access to the subclavian artery.

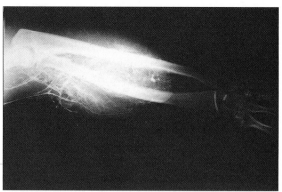

5.28 Crush injury to the forearm. A severe crush injury, as seen here, may result in acute ischaemia. In this case, pulses were absent at the wrist and arteriography showed bleeding into the proximal forearm and no visible distal large arteries. Emergency exploration was required.

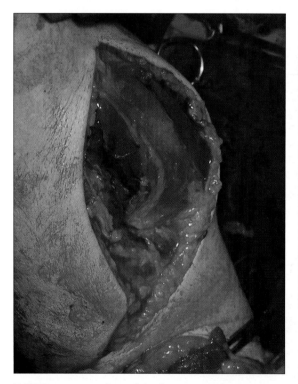

5.29 Decompression of the forearm. A large haematoma under the deep fascia, which had completely occluded the distal arm circulation, was revealed on decompressing the forearm. Relief of the compression immediately restored distal perfusion.

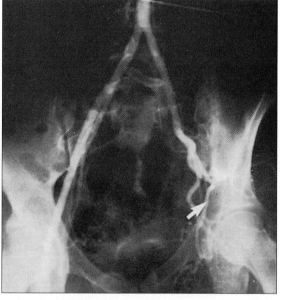

5.30 Cardiac catheterization. One of the commonest iatrogenic causes of acute limb ischaemia is femoral arterial puncture. The ischaemia usually results from the raising of a subintimal flap followed by thrombosis of the vessel (arrow). Smaller modern catheters have dramatically reduced, but not eliminated, the overall incidence of catheter-associated problems. In this case, the left femoral artery was catheterized for coronary arteriography. Excessive bleeding necessitated open suture of the artery by the cardiologist, which was followed by thrombosis of the artery as seen here.

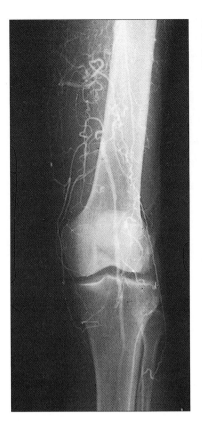

5.31 Arterial damage due to catheters. This is most likely to occur when the brachial artery is used for cannulation. In this case injury to the artery at the elbow has resulted in thrombosis of the entire brachial artery. For this reason, the brachial artery is not generally favoured for arterial catheter access.

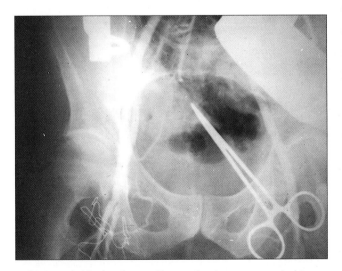

5.32 Arterial intimal tear. This can be due to surgery. In this case, an aorto–bifemoral bypass was inserted into the common femoral arteries. Poor distal pulses were found and an 'on-table' angiogram was performed. This shows a tight stenosis at the origin of the superficial artery on the right. Exploration revealed an intimal flap, which required tacking down in order to obtain a satisfactory result.

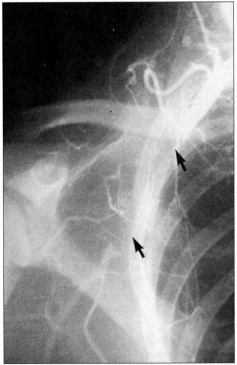

5.33 Hyperextension injury of the shoulder. Arterial damage can result from a hyperextension injury of the shoulder without any obvious external signs of injury. This motor cycle rider had 'come off' his bike and sustained a brachial plexus avulsion injury without laceration. Axillary artery thrombosis (arrows) was demonstrated on the angiogram.

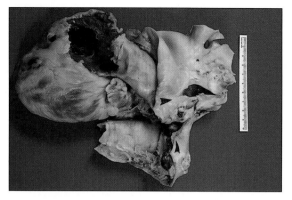

5.34 Rupture of the aortic arch. This injury occurs in association with severe deceleration, such as occurs in a severe road traffic accident. The two points where rupture is most often found are at the aortic root and at the left subclavian artery. In this case, rupture has occurred at both points and also involved the right ventricle. Death was instantaneous. Emergency angiography is required if there is a suspicion of aortic injury after any severe accident. Plain chest radiographic findings include widening of the mediastinum, a pleural effusion in the left chest and tracheal shift.

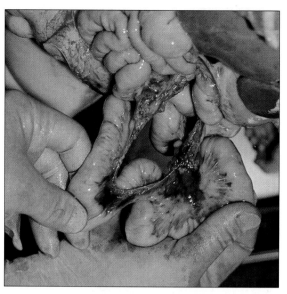

5.35 Rupture of mesenteric vessels. Blunt injury to the abdomen, such as from a seat belt, can cause tearing of the mesentery, as here, where the torn vessels resulted in the death of this child.

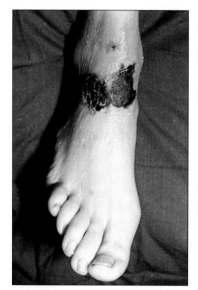

5.36 Acute ischaemia due to pressure necrosis from a plaster of Paris. This should never occur if the plaster is put on properly, bivalved and a careful plaster check performed, particularly when the injury is fresh and swelling is to be expected. Failure to abide by these rules may lead to a disastrous outcome, as seen here.

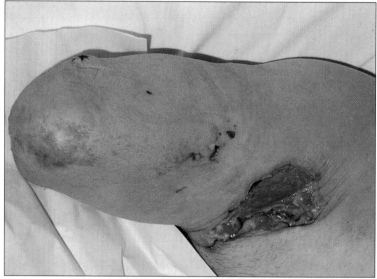

5.37 Excessive tight bandaging. This may also be a cause of acute ischaemia. In this case, the damage is confined to local skin necrosis.

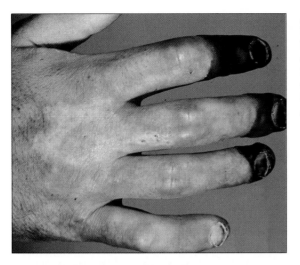

5.38 Chemical-induced arterial thrombosis. The intra-arterial injection of various noxious substances is increasingly seen in major city casualty departments. One drug that is commonly used in this way is temazepam, which induces a particularly severe microthrombosis that often threatens the viability of the involved limb, usually the arm. Urgent treatment with heparin and intravenous prostacyclin or analogues will dramatically reduce the degree of damage in such cases. The hand of a drug addict who inadvertently injected his brachial artery is shown here.

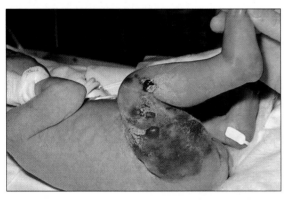

5.39 Iatrogenic chemical arterial injury. A toxic substance was inadvertently injected into the umbilical artery of this baby. Fortunately, the effect was limited to the skin of the upper thigh.

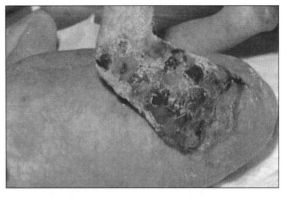

5.40 Skin grafting. In this case, skin grafting was required after demarcation and sloughing of the necrotic area.

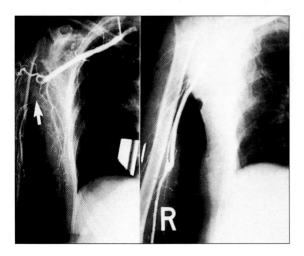

5.41 Irradiation arterial damage. A less common cause of arterial occlusion is radiation therapy. Excessive exposure of the arterial wall to such treatment induces an acute inflammatory reaction, which on occasion can lead to thrombosis. In other cases, such as that seen here, a more gradual progression of occlusive disease may be seen due to fibrosis in the arterial wall. This post-mastectomy patient developed occlusion of the proximal brachial artery and required a vein bypass as seen here on the right.

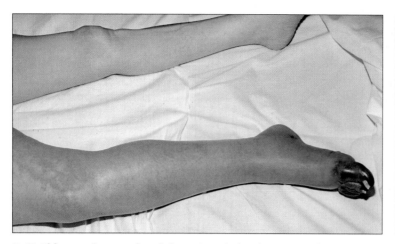

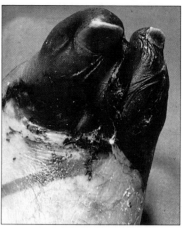

5.42 Phlegmasia caerulea dolens. Acute limb ischaemia may have an underlying venous cause, as here, where congestion and limb swelling with or without secondary arterial thrombosis produces marked ischaemia leading to gangrene. Note the gross swelling and dusky appearance, which suggests a primary venous problem. In this case, venous thrombectomy was performed to relieve the situation with a successful outcome, although in many cases thrombosis will re-occur despite apparently successful venous thrombectomy.

5.43 Severe venous gangrene secondary to bilateral deep venous thrombosis. This patient has an underlying carcinoma of the pancreas. Aggressive heparinization and elevation of the limb may prevent this extending more proximally, but the prognosis for the patient is obviously poor.

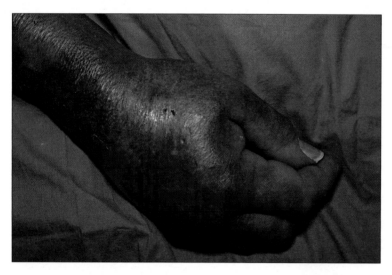

5.44 Acute axillary vein thrombosis. This is not always a benign entity. In this case the venous occlusion has been sufficient to cause necrosis of the hand. Pulmonary embolism is also possible with upper limb venous thrombosis and most patients should be systemically anticoagulated when diagnosed.

6.
Chronic Occlusive Vascular Disease

Occlusive arterial disease is a progressive process of developing stenoses and acute-on-chronic occlusions in the major and medium-sized arteries. Its effects are most noticeable in the heart, cerebrovascular circulation and lower limbs, although it may affect any or all of the arteries in the body. The common clinical symptoms are therefore angina, myocardial infarction, stroke, claudication and critical ischaemia of the lower limbs. The presence, exact presentation and severity of symptoms depend upon many factors, but especially important are the precise site of the stenosis or occlusion and the rapidity of onset of the lesion.

LOWER LIMB DISEASE

The main site of arterial stenosis or occlusion is the superficial femoral artery, usually at the adductor hiatus, with the principal symptom being calf claudication. The disease is often bilateral, although symptoms may be confined to the worst side. In claudication patients, one or more pulses may be diminished or absent in the leg. Where pulses are felt in the feet, a bruit may be detectable over the adductor canal after a short period of exercise, suggesting stenotic disease in the superficial femoral artery.

Critical limb ischaemia (CLI) is the term used to describe a limb that is 'threatened' (i.e. major amputation will probably be required in the absence of intervention). In practice, many patients defined as having 'critical' ischaemia are actually 'subcritical' in that they do not have an immediate risk of limb loss. The presenting symptom of a patient with true CLI is therefore gangrene, ulceration or severe rest pain. Generally, an ankle pressure of less than 50 mmHg or a toe pressure of less than 30 mmHg is required to be definitive about the diagnosis, but many cases of true CLI fall outside this rather artificial definition.

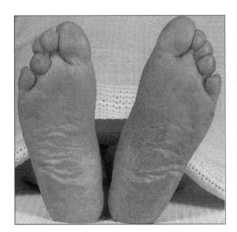

6.1 Intermittent claudication. The soles of the feet are observed with the patient lying flat. Often no significant difference will be seen, but in this patient, the right foot is slightly paler than the left. The patient presented with calf claudication at about 100 m.

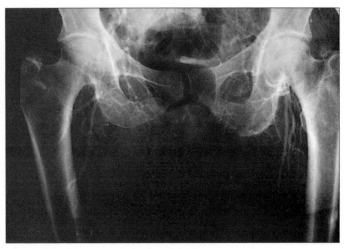

6.2 Thigh and sometimes buttock claudication. This is seen if the common femoral artery is occluded, in this case on both sides. If the profunda femoral artery also becomes involved, severe symptoms are likely, and critical ischaemia is possible.

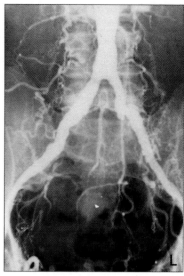

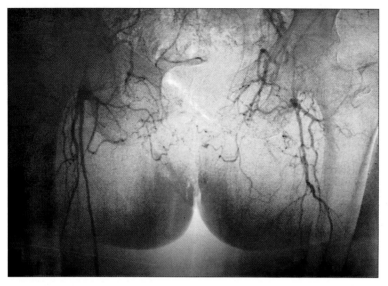

6.3 Subtraction views of femoral occlusion. In some cases, digital subtraction images may give a clearer view of the level of involvement and degree of collateralization.

6.4 Common iliac stenosis. This is a common finding in patients with middle distance claudication. Clinically, this patient had a reduced left femoral pulse and a left iliac bruit.

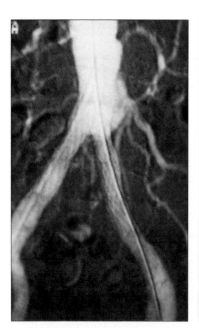

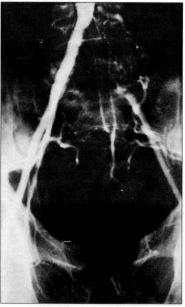

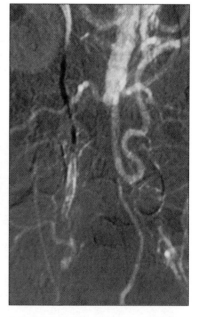

6.5 Iliac angioplasty. The best method of dealing with common iliac stenosis is by percutaneous transluminal angioplasty. Nowadays, many of these lesions are stented (as here) to maintain the lumen and reduce the incidence of re-stenosis, which is high with angioplasty.

6.6 Common iliac occlusion. Although traditionally patients with these lesions used to be offered surgical correction, percutaneous recanalization angioplasty with or without stenting is possible in most cases and has good long-term results.

6.7 Complete occlusion of the aorta. In some patients, it is possible for the entire infrarenal aorta to occlude over a period. If the occlusion is gradual, there may be remarkably few symptoms. In this case, however, the patient complained of buttock and thigh claudication in association with impotence—the Leriche syndrome.

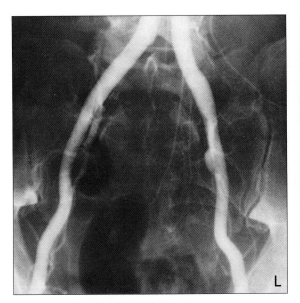

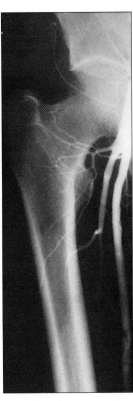

6.9 Superficial femoral artery stenosis. The commonest point at which significant arterial lesions are seen in peripheral vascular disease is at the adductor hiatus. In many cases, such lesions may be suitable for angioplasty, but there is some evidence that a properly coordinated exercise programme combined with a modification of risk factors (especially smoking) may offer a medium- and long-term outlook as good as, if not better than, that provided by angioplasty.

6.8 Internal iliac occlusion. In this case, the patient complained of impotence and buttock claudication. Angiography shows that the left internal iliac artery is occluded and the right internal iliac artery is severely diseased. Although it is tempting to attribute the patient's impotence to vascular insufficiency, most cases of impotence are not due to vascular disease.

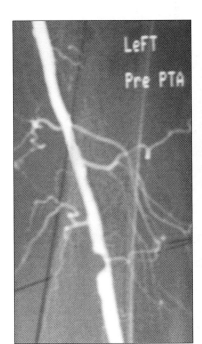

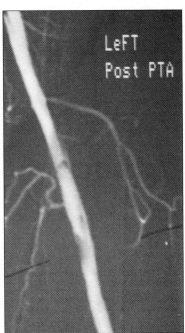

6.10 Angioplasty of superficial femoral artery stenosis. Successful angioplasty has been completed here and ankle pressure has returned to normal. To date, the use of intraluminal stents in the superficial femoral artery has not increased patency rates overall and cannot be justified in view of their high cost.

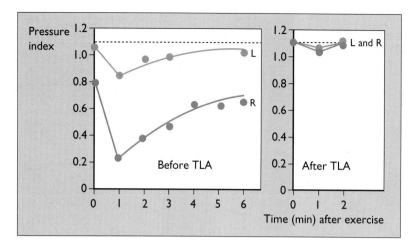

6.11 Doppler pressure studies before and after angioplasty. Here the results of angioplasty can be graphically seen with the response to exercise testing. Following angioplasty, the right leg has regained a near-normal performance.

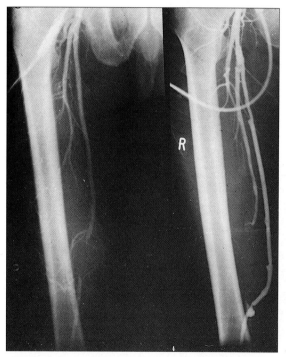

6.12 Short superficial femoral artery occlusion. This used to be treated with local bypass, as shown here. Now, the treatment would be recanalization angioplasty, which when used for appropriate (short) lesions produces results comparable to those of bypass at 1 year (70–80% patency rates). Although much research has been carried out into the use of laser recanalization and atherectomy devices, there is no long-term evidence that they offer any improvement in outcome over that resulting from a well-performed percutaneous angioplasty alone.

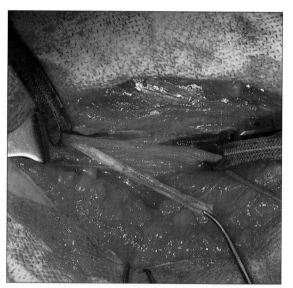

6.13 Superficial femoral endarterectomy. This operation was much favoured in the past, but has fallen into disrepute because of unacceptably high failure rates and restenosis problems. Here the artery has been opened out and a core of atheroma removed. The artery is then usually patched to widen the resultant lumen.

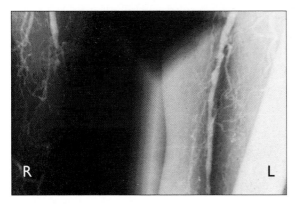

6.14 Long superficial femoral artery occlusion.
Many patients with short to middle distance calf claudication
have complete occlusion of the superficial femoral artery, as
here. This group of patients is perhaps the hardest to
manage because they are unsuitable for percutaneous
angioplasty and yet their symptoms are worse than those of
patients who may be offered angioplasty. Except in specific
cases, most vascular surgeons are reluctant to embark on
femoro–popliteal bypass. Therefore, the majority of these
patients are inevitably offered conservative management.

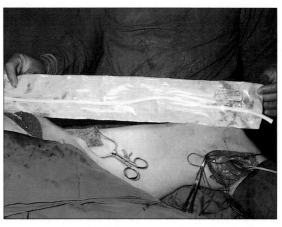

6.15 Femoro–popliteal bypass. In some patients,
claudication is so severe that it drastically reduces their
quality of life. In selected cases leg bypass may be
considered using a femoro–popliteal bypass, as here. It is
important to inform the patient that at least 20% of grafts
may not be functioning at 1 year and to ensure that all risk
factors have been addressed, with a special emphasis on
stopping smoking.

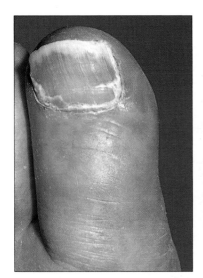

6.16 Blue toe syndrome. This is
quite a common presentation in
vascular outpatients and is usually due
to microembolization from disease in
the superficial femoral artery. It can,
however, result from any proximal
source of thrombosis/embolism. In this
case, a stenosis of the superficial
femoral artery was found. Successful
angioplasty dramatically relieved the
discoloration.

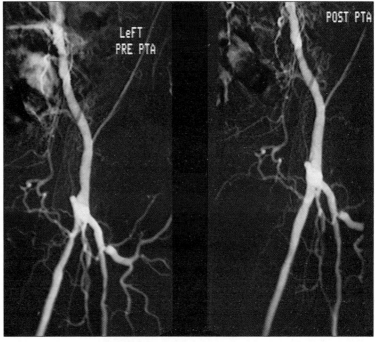

6.17 Proximal graft stenosis. This patient had a previous femoro–popliteal
bypass graft for short-distance intermittent claudication. Nine months after the
operation, he complained of further claudication and angiography revealed a
stenosis at the top end of the graft. This was successfully treated by angioplasty,
with complete relief of his symptoms, as shown on the right of the picture.

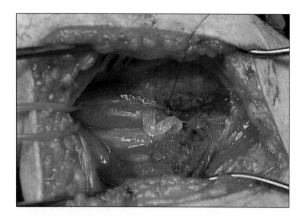

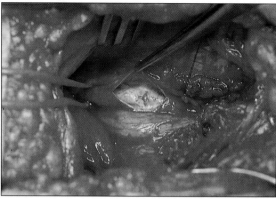

6.18 Popliteal adventitial cyst. This young man presented with intermittent claudication that prevented him from hill-walking. Angiography revealed a severe atypical stenosis in his popliteal artery, which was explored. A popliteal adventitial cyst was found. The gelatinous material can be seen exuding through a small incision in the adventitia.

6.19 Popliteal adventitial cyst. The cyst contents seen in **6.18** has now been completely cleared and the integrity of the lumen retained. Following excision of the cyst wall, the ankle pressures returned to normal and the claudication symptoms resolved.

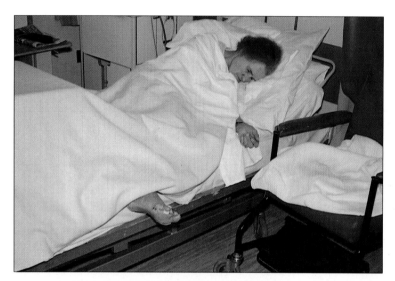

6.20 Rest pain. One of the commonest manifestations of CLI is rest pain. This is pain in the toes or forefoot that has been present for at least 2 weeks and is a consequence of arterial insufficiency. It is worse when lying horizontal (as at night) and will classically keep the patient awake or wake him or her up. It may be temporarily relieved by hanging the limb over the edge of the bed, as seen here, or by standing up and (paradoxically) taking a few steps around the room. Ultimately, dependent oedema from persistent limb dependency will worsen the microcirculation and probably lead to necrosis.

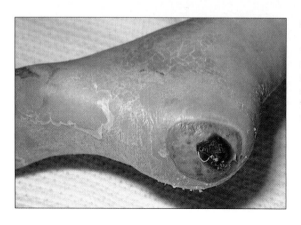

6.21 Pressure sore. A common cause of skin breakdown in the elderly is prolonged enforced bedrest with a failure to relieve pressure areas such as the heel, as seen here. Skin necrosis and ulceration is more likely if the arterial circulation is compromised, but may occur in the presence of a normal circulation. It is important to look for evidence of vascular disease when assessing such patients because in many cases healing may be impossible without intervention.

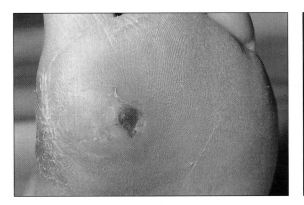

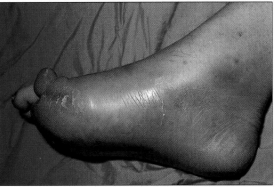

6.22 Diabetic ulcer. This patient has a typical diabetic neurotrophic ulcer over the head of the metatarsals. Most of these patients can be adequately treated with conservative management and some will benefit enormously from a plaster of Paris slipper to protect the foot and ulcer. Occasionally local excision is required. The best management is of course prevention, and all diabetic patients should be counselled about foot care and advised to attend a good chiropodist.

6.23 Osteomyelitis. In some diabetic patients local infection may mimic ischaemia and it can be difficult to discriminate one from the other initially. This patient was admitted as an emergency with 'critical ischaemia' to the vascular unit. Careful examination revealed a swollen, warm foot with exquisite tenderness over the first metatarsal head. In addition, there was significant limb ischaemia. A bone scan confirmed the clinical impression of osteomyelitis and local excision of the bone with aggressive antibiotics salvaged the foot without recourse to revascularization.

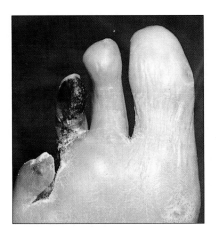

6.24 Chronic ischaemic ulceration. This patient had a long history of occlusive arterial disease and had had previous digital amputation. On this occasion, he presented with digital gangrene and severe rest pain, necessitating a distal bypass. Many patients with severe peripheral vascular disease will re-present in the following months and years for further management because of the progressive nature of the illness.

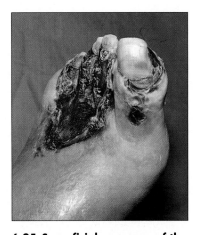

6.25 Superficial gangrene of the toes. It is important to assess as accurately as possible the extent of local foot gangrene. In this case, the necrosis, though quite extensive, is largely superficial, and following reconstruction only digital amputations were required.

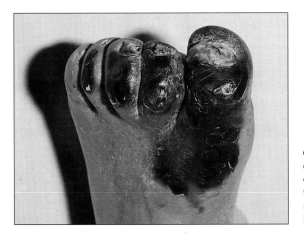

6.26 Deep gangrene of the forefoot. Although apparently similar to that shown in **6.25**, this patient had deep gangrene of the distal forefoot extending through to the plantar surface. Following revascularization, a trans-metatarsal amputation of the forefoot was required to allow healing to take place.

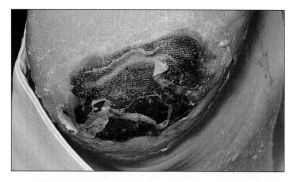

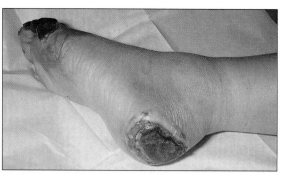

6.27 Ischaemic heel necrosis. This is often precipitated by prolonged bedrest. It is important to ascertain the extent of tissue involvement because a superficial necrosis is likely to heal following revascularization, as here, but it is difficult to achieve healing of deep necrosis involving the calcaneum or the Achilles tendon, even if the blood supply has been well restored.

6.28 Ischaemic heel necrosis (deep). If the necrosis is deep seated, and particularly if there is extensive gangrene elsewhere, as here, it may be wiser to elect for a primary transtibial amputation, which allows definitive management and a much quicker rehabilitation and mobilization.

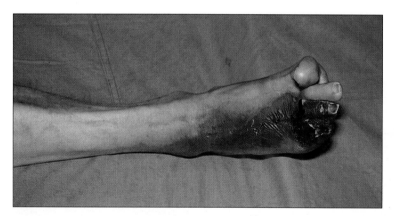

6.29 Extensive foot necrosis. Where the hind foot is involved with gangrene, there is no point in attempting reconstructive vascular surgery and primary amputation should be performed. Wherever possible, this should be carried out at the transtibial (below-knee) level because the chances of successful mobilization with a prosthesis are much greater.

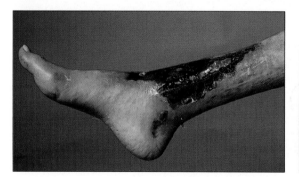

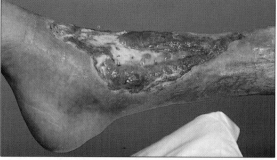

6.30 Iatrogenic ulceration. This patient fractured his ankle and had an open reduction and plating by the orthopaedic surgeons. Unfortunately, he had a marginal preoperative arterial flow to the foot and this was not recognized. His wound subsequently broke down, exposing the plate and tibia. It is important to search for pulses in all patients who are about to undergo distal limb surgery. If there is any doubt, Doppler pressure studies should be performed and, if necessary, arteriography.

6.31 Iatrogenic ulceration post-revascularization. It was possible to salvage the limb of the patient shown in **6.30** by performing a femoro–peroneal bypass to the mid-peroneal artery, which was exposed by excising a short length of fibula. Excellent reperfusion was achieved to the foot and, after excision of dead tissue and removal of the plate, granulation tissue rapidly filled in the defect as seen here 10 days later. Secondary skin grafting achieved a most satisfactory outcome.

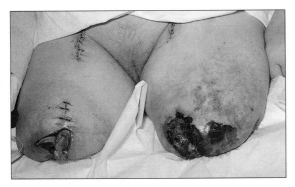

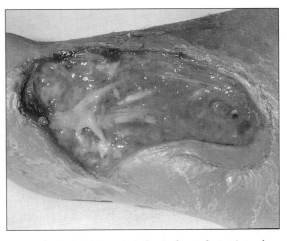

6.32 Above-knee amputation stump necrosis. This lady was admitted with bilateral stump necrosis 6 weeks after amputation for occlusive vascular disease without preliminary vascular assessment. On admission, she was taking 400 mg morphine per day and clinical examination revealed no femoral pulses. An emergency axillo–biprofunda bypass was performed without angiography and despite the obviously truncated distal profunda, this worked very well. Sadly, despite a vastly improved thigh circulation, the patient died 2 weeks later from pneumonia, presumably exacerbated by the prolonged high opiate dosages.

6.33 Local excision of diabetic foot ulceration. If there is local ulceration in a diabetic foot with necrosis, it may be possible to excise the area and expect healing, unlike in atherosclerotic occlusive vascular disease. Here, extensive debridement has been performed and granulation tissue is evident in the base of the wound. Careful aftercare with a plaster of Paris slipper allowed complete healing.

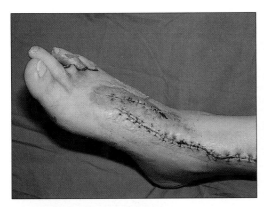

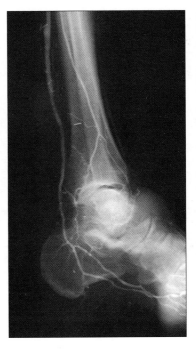

6.34 Dorsalis pedis bypass. In some patients with very severe vascular disease, only a bypass to the foot is possible, as here, where a femoro–dorsalis pedis bypass has been achieved with an *in situ* vein technique. A concomitant third toe amputation was also required. The foot healed and rest pain was relieved for 2 years until the patient's death. It is important to remember that patients with CLI have a limited life expectancy (much less than patients with a Duke's B carcinoma of the colon).

6.35 Posterior tibial bypass. Here the post-operative angiogram shows a distal vein bypass to the posterior tibial artery at the ankle. The surgical clips used and the peroneal artery can be seen. Although it may have been possible to bypass to a more proximal peroneal artery, this does not communicate directly to the foot and if there is gangrene it is probably best to use the posterior tibial or anterior tibial vessels if one of these is present.

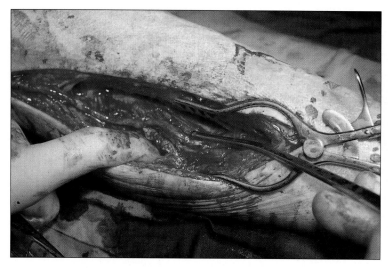

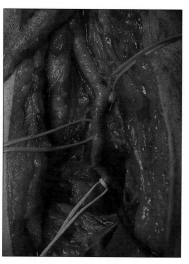

6.36 Peroneal artery bypass. Here, a vein bypass has been performed to the mid-peroneal artery in the calf. This may be approached either laterally by excising a short length of fibula or medially, as here. It is one of the more difficult dissections to perform because the artery is deep-lying and invariably surrounded by a plexus of collateral veins. Although only communicating with the foot via its anterior and posterior perforating branches, it is frequently the only remaining tibial vessel available for bypass. In practice, it offers excellent outflow because of its numerous muscular branches.

6.37 Profunda femoris artery exploration. The profunda femoral artery is the key to limb survival in many cases. However, it is often necessary to dissect out the middle and even distal thirds of the vessel in order to get a good lumen. Here the profunda femoral artery and its branches are displayed before an extensive endarterectomy and patch.

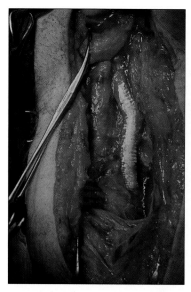

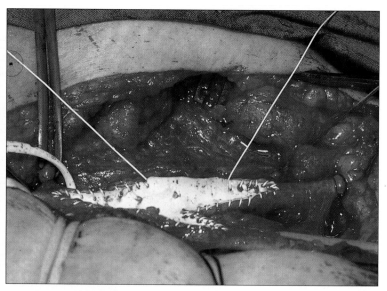

6.38 Profunda femoral artery patch angioplasty. The femoral artery has been closed with a PTFE patch after endarterectomy and a good technical result has been achieved here.

6.39 Patch angioplasty. In many cases, a local profundaplasty with a patch is sufficient to increase blood flow to the limb and to alleviate rest pain. Here a PTFE patch is customized to allow flow down both the profunda and superficial femoral vessels.

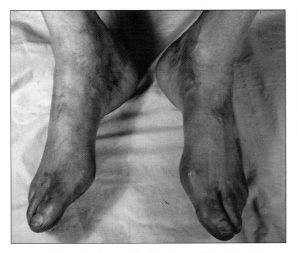

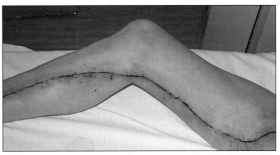

6.41 Distal leg bypass–skin scar. When a distal bypass is required, the long saphenous vein is the conduit of choice and it is generally necessary to expose it throughout most of its length, as here. Although this wound is healing well, up to 25% of long distal bypass wounds will have problems, usually in the form of skin edge necrosis and superficial infection. This adds considerably to the patient's stay in hospital and discomfort.

6.40 Bilateral microembolization of the feet. This man presented with a several-week history of pain and coldness in his feet. Examination revealed severe bilateral discoloration of the feet and barely palpable pedal pulses, and in addition, he was noted to have an aortic aneurysm. This is a case of embolization from an aortic aneurysm. Where signs are bilateral, as here, it is likely that the problem is proximal to the aortic bifurcation. If the signs are unilateral, then the source is more likely to arise from the iliac, femoral or popliteal arteries.

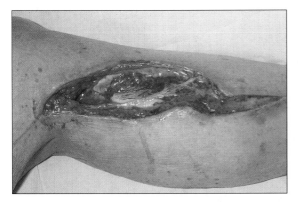

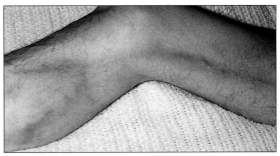

6.42 Wound breakdown. Here a distal bypass wound has broken down due to skin edge necrosis and has been formally debrided and left open. Fortunately, in this case the vein graft is to the peroneal artery and lies deep to the muscle at this point, reducing the chance of a secondary haemorrhage.

6.43 Vascular surgeon's nightmare! Here, the long saphenous vein has thrombosed and the vein can be seen outlined with superficial thrombophebitis, rendering it useless as a bypass. In these cases, vein may be harvested from the other leg or the arms; on occasions it is possible to use the short saphenous and superficial femoral veins, generally as composite vein bypasses. However, this makes revascularization of the limb a very long operation and some surgeons will opt for a PTFE graft even though the medium- and long-term results are poor.

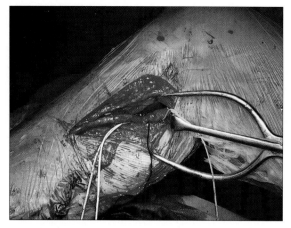

6.44 Popliteal–pedal bypass. Many patients, especially diabetics, have good flow to the popliteal artery. In these patients, it is possible to use the popliteal artery for the proximal anastomosis, as here. This requires a shorter bypass and a shorter length of healthy vein, both of which are desirable.

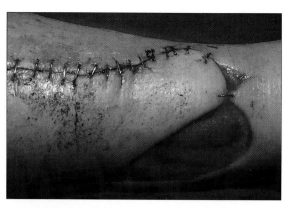

6.45 Rotation skin flap. Occasionally it may be necessary to cover the distal anastomosis with healthy skin, as here. This patient had an infected distal bypass that required revision. This was revised with a distal vein graft repair and a rotation skin flap covered the region. A split skin graft was used to cover the resultant defect and this allowed complete healing with a patent graft at 1-year follow-up.

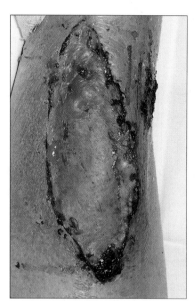

6.46 Split skin graft. Occasionally a split skin graft is required to cover a distal wound if there is considerable leg swelling and thin skin, as here. This skin graft covered a femoro–anterior tibial distal graft site and healed well.

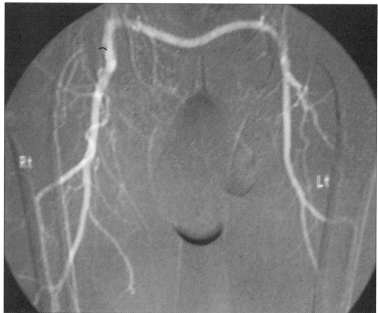

6.47 Femoro–femoral crossover graft. Angiograph showing the postoperative appearance of a femoro-femoral crossover graft. Note that the graft is running from right to left and is placed into the proximal profunda femoris artery.

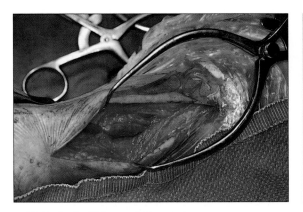

6.48 Technical hiccough! Surgical expertise is important in performing distal bypass grafting. In this case, the tunnelled portion of an anterior tibial bypass to the ankle was inadvertently twisted through 360°, resulting in the twist appearing at the distal anastomosis when flow was established. This slightly embarrassing defect was easily remedied by division and re-anastomosis of the vein graft at the site of the twist. Postoperative 'on-table' angiography is highly desirable to eliminate any technical errors and to maximize the chances of a successful distal bypass.

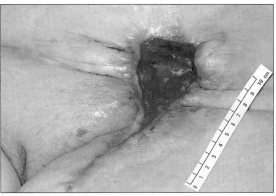

6.49 Groin wound sepsis. A major problem in vascular surgery is the healing of groin wounds, especially after revisional vascular surgery. Infection in such wounds may be disastrous and result in a graft infection with subsequent loss of limb and even life.

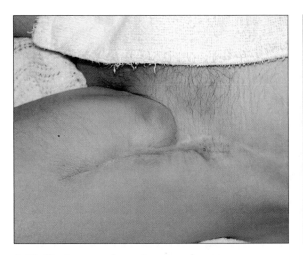

6.50 Groin wound sepsis—pseudoaneurysm. Another complication of groin sepsis is the development of an infected anastomosis and subsequent pseudoaneurysm formation, as here. Surgery for this is complicated and difficult.

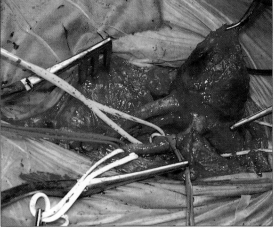

6.51 Revisional surgery. This remains the most challenging aspect of vascular disease from a technical viewpoint. Because many patients return with blocked grafts or further disease progression, it is important to become familiar with the techniques of secondary revascularization. Here, a pseudoaneurysm from a previous occluded femoro–popliteal bypass has been dissected out, along with the common, superficial and profunda femoral arteries.

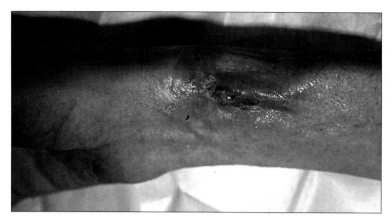

6.52 Infected Cimino arteriovenous fistula. Infection may occur in any area of the body, but is most likely where repeated invasion of the skin is performed, as in renal dialysis. Here a radio–cephalic fistula has become grossly infected and at this stage is probably beyond salvage.

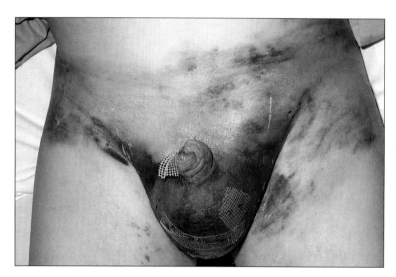

6.53 Haemorrhage after arteriogram. This illustration shows extensive bruising secondary to a bleed following coronary catheterization. Such haemorrhage is now relatively rare because of the use of small-bore catheters, but does occasionally occur, particularly if there is common femoral artery disease, which makes vessel wall tearing more likely. Despite this, day-case and even outpatient angiography is now a relatively safe procedure.

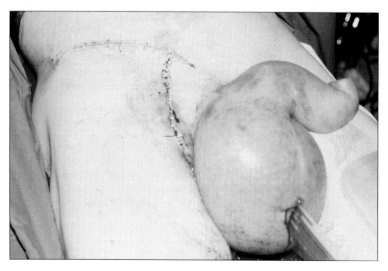

6.54 Haemorrhage following attempted thrombolysis. Here a cannula was placed into the distal external iliac artery for thrombolysis. The patient subsequently bled profusely into his retroperitoneum and had to be taken to theatre as an emergency. Scrotal decompression was required. All thrombolysis cannulas should be placed directly into the common femoral artery so that any bleeding is visible and compression is easily applied.

AMPUTATION

Despite the advances in limb salvage, a large number of patients still require major limb amputation for end-stage peripheral vascular disease. The ultimate functional result and quality of life for the patient depends largely on the expertise of the amputating surgeon, the level of amputation and the rehabilitation facilities available.

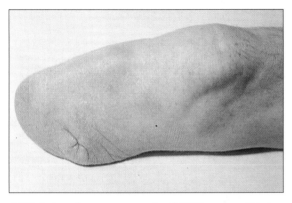

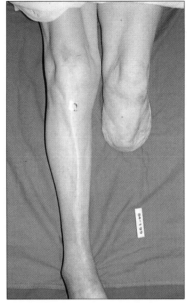

6.56 Contralateral ischaemia. This patient who has a healed left BKA now presents with a critically ischaemic right leg. About 20% of amputees ultimately lose their contralateral leg.

6.55 Below-knee amputation (BKA) stump. This is a good example of a healed BKA or transtibial amputation stump. Patients with BKA stumps are far more likely to achieve independence and to walk than those who have an above-knee (AKA) or transfemoral amputation.

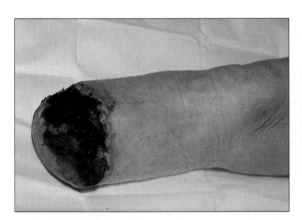

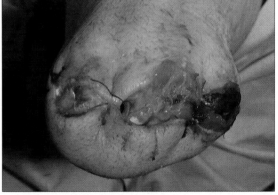

6.57 Below-knee stump breakdown. This is the reason that many surgeons cite for not attempting BKAs. However, such a result must be seen as a failure of technique, either in determining the level of amputation or of operative technique. It should be possible to achieve BKA:AKA ratios of more than 2:1 in any vascular unit.

6.58 Bad amputation surgery. Here the amputation was left to an inexperienced junior surgeon who has used a poor technique and large tight skin sutures, resulting in stump breakdown and sepsis. Amputation surgery should be performed by or supervised by the most experienced surgeon available in the unit.

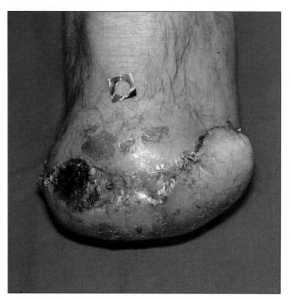

6.59 Below-knee stump ischaemia. The lateral edge of this stump has necrosed. However, a local wedge resection salvaged this as a good below-knee stump. In many cases it is the lateral edge that is most vunerable due to the relatively poorer skin blood flow in this area.

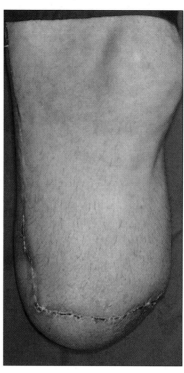

6.60 Healed below-knee amputation after failed distal bypass. Although it has been suggested that an aggressive revascularization will result in more AKAs, this has not happened, although there is a relative reduction in the ratio of BKA:AKA. Distal (tibial) bypasses do not normally interfere with the geniculate anastomoses around the knee and therefore do not generally prejudice the outcome of any subsequent BKA.

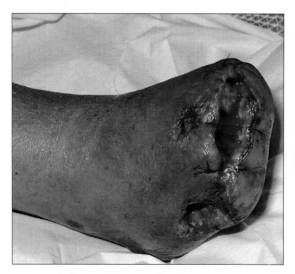

6.61 Failed transmetatarsal amputation. Foot and most digital amputations will not heal in the absence of adequate revascularization unless there is purely a microvascular problem, as is found in some insulin-dependent diabetics. This is an example of an ill-advised attempt to resect distal gangrene without revascularization.

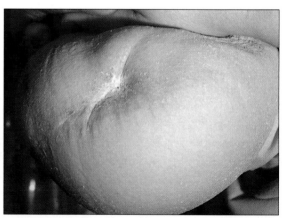

6.62 High above-knee amputation. In some cases, an AKA has to be carried out as a life-saving measure. Here the patient presented with an occluded femoro–popliteal graft and an occluded common femoral artery, which was left too late to salvage. High AKA eventually healed after prolonged hospitalization, but the patient's subsequent mobility was dependent upon a wheelchair. It is often difficult to adequately mobilize the elderly patient with such a stump.

7.
Cerebrovascular Disease and Disease of the Thoracic Aorta

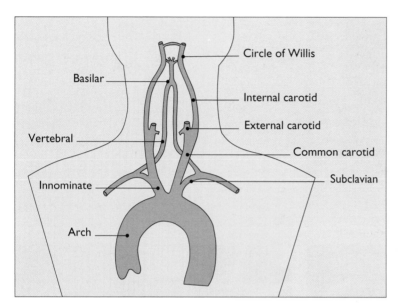

7.1 Arterial blood supply to the brain. This schematic diagram shows the arterial blood supply to the brain. The outlined figure does not show the exact division of the vessels. Although occlusions, either single or multiple, can influence the blood supply to the brain, the main extracranial source of symptoms is thought to be embolization of debris from the carotid bifurcation, which may result in a transient ischaemic attack (TIA) or a stroke.

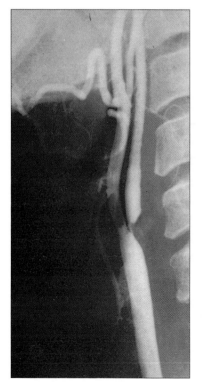

7.2 High-grade stenosis of the carotid artery. Angiography here demonstrates a very tight (at least 95%) stenosis of the right internal carotid artery at the bifurcation. Such a lesion is very likely to be due to a heterogeneous plaque, which may embolize, giving rise to cerebrovascular symptoms. Invariably, a carotid bruit will be heard, although this can be absent in particularly tight lesions. When the lesion is symptomatic and over 70% stenosed, studies have shown that surgery confers the best chance of avoiding a subsequent ipsilateral hemispheric stroke.

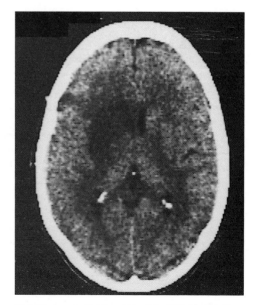

7.3 Computed tomographic (CT) scan of the brain. For many patients presenting with TIAs, it is useful to perform a CT scan of the brain. In some, as here, a cerebral infarct will be seen, and there may be a similar finding in some patients with 'asymptomatic' carotid artery stenosis.

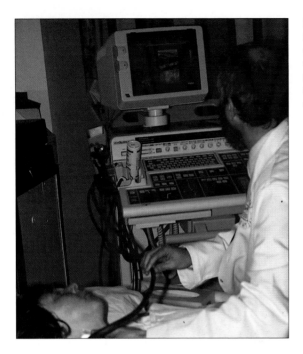

7.4 Duplex scanning of the carotid vessels. This is now regarded as the gold standard investigation for extracranial cerebrovascular disease in patients presenting with a stroke, a TIA, amaurosis fugax, nonspecific symptoms or asymptomatic carotid artery bruits. Many centres now avoid angiography altogether and are prepared to operate on the basis of ultrasound findings alone.

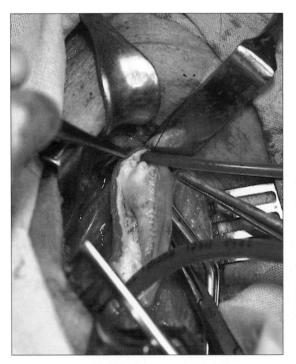

7.5 Carotid endarterectomy. The common, external and internal carotid arteries are clearly seen following endarterectomy of the plaque. When performing carotid surgery, it is advisable to avoid handling (and therefore not to dissect out) the bifurcation until distal control of the internal carotid artery has been achieved by clamping. This reduces the risk of embolization from the plaque in the artery, which should be treated with the same respect as a grenade!

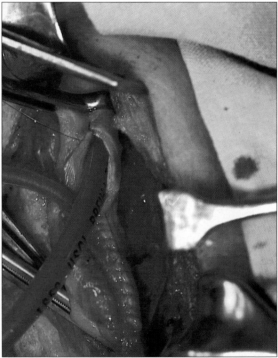

7.6 Carotid endarterectomy. Here, the common and internal carotid arteries are being closed with a vein patch. A temporary indwelling shunt (Javid-type) is in place to allow continuous blood flow to the hemisphere. There is, however, no proven difference in perioperative stroke rates between shunted and non-shunted patients, although the use of a shunt usually makes the surgeon feel more comfortable.

CAROTID PLAQUE MORPHOLOGY

Because of the probability that carotid plaques are a major source of embolization, it has been suggested that compound ulcerated plaques with thrombosis and instability may be more likely to result in cerebrovascular symptoms. Plaques are therefore classified as follows and may be described on Duplex scanning preoperatively.

- Type I: Almost exclusively haemorrhagic plaque with intraplaque disruption and debris; echolucent on B-mode ultrasound.

- Type II: Predominantly haemorrhagic, but with some fibrous elements suggesting remodelling.
- Type III: Largely fibrous plaque, but with some compound features.
- Type IV: Almost exclusively fibrous plaque with no evidence of heterogeneity; highly echogenic on ultrasound.

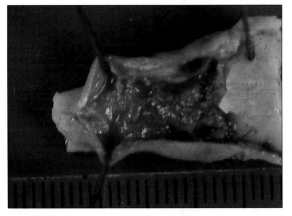

7.7 Carotid plaque. This is an example of an endarterectomy specimen from a carotid bifurcation. This is a Type I plaque with predominantly haemorrhagic features and made up of a large amount of clot and loose debris. It can be immediately appreciated why such a plaque is considered to be dangerous in the cerebrovascular blood flow. Type I plaques are much more likely to be associated with a high-grade (> 70%) stenosis.

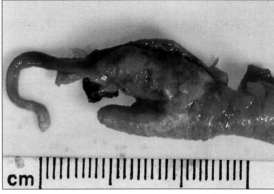

7.8 Occlusion of the internal carotid artery. This endarterectomy specimen was taken from a patient who had an occluded internal carotid artery. Despite the theoretical benefit from improved blood flow with surgery, studies have not shown any clinical benefit from surgery in such patients, underlining the role of embolization as the main cause of cerebrovascular symptoms. Once the internal carotid artery is occluded, embolization is very unlikely, although clearly a low-flow situation may exist and give rise to symptoms.

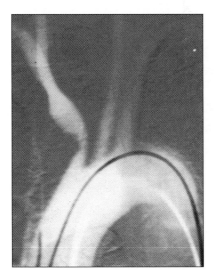

7.9 Innominate artery stenosis. In some cases, the carotid artery is not responsible for cerebral emboli. Here, a duplex scan suggested a low flow proximal to the common carotid artery. Angiography was performed, revealing a stenosis of the innominate artery, which was easily repaired with an aorto–innominate bypass, with subsequent resolution of the symptoms. Nowadays, such lesions are increasingly treated with percutaneous transluminal angioplasty. Although there is a theoretical risk from embolization at angioplasty, this has not proved to be a major problem in the small series described to date.

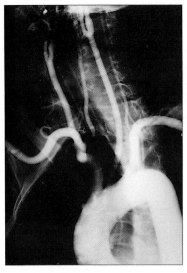

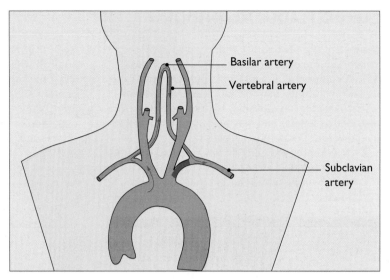

7.10 Vertebral artery stenosis.
This may cause less specific symptomatology such as 'drop attacks' due to posterior cerebral/cerebellar ischaemia. However, most such attacks are not due to cerebrovascular ischaemia and great care should be taken when making this diagnosis. This illustration shows bilateral vertebral artery stenosis. Generally, there is an associated carotid artery stenosis, as seen here.

7.11 Vertebrobasilar insufficiency. A complete block of the proximal subclavian artery can lead to a subclavian steal syndrome in which there is a reversed flow in the ipsilateral vertebral artery due to an increased demand for flow in the upper limb after exercise. This syndrome may be seen with either angiography or Duplex scanning.

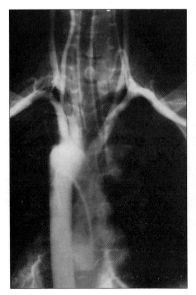

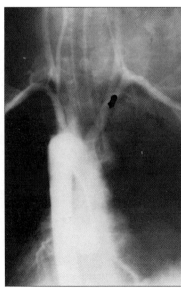

7.12 Stenosis of the subclavian artery. This usually occurs near the origin of the subclavian artery and may present with claudication in the affected arm or occasionally subclavian steal syndrome. More usually, however, it is a common incidental finding. The pulse will be reduced on the affected side and the arm systolic pressure less than on the other side. In the left picture, an atheromatous plaque is present in the right subclavian artery. In the right picture, the removed plaque is superimposed upon the angiogram.

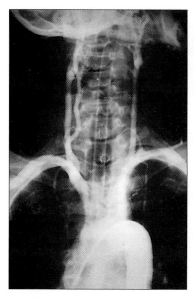

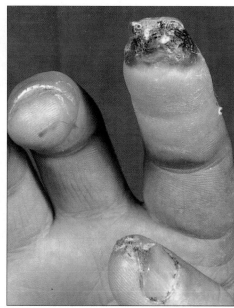

7.14 Digital gangrene from subclavian embolus. A stenosis of the right subclavian artery was found to be responsible for the emboli to this man's index finger and thumb. He had initially presented with what was thought to be unilateral Raynaud's phenomenon.

7.13 Stenosis of the left vertebral artery. This stenosis is easily seen here; however, the associated severe stenosis of the left subclavian artery is not so easily visualized, being somewhat obscured by the left clavicle. The right vertebral artery is clearly seen and is normal.

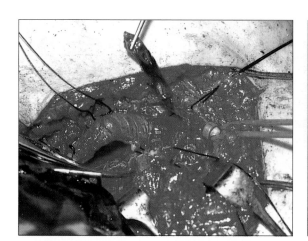

7.15 Subclavian artery thrombosis. Here, the artery has been stretched over an underlying cervical rib. The artery has been opened and the thrombus is being removed. Part of such a thrombus could easily embolize distally to the hand or digital vessels.

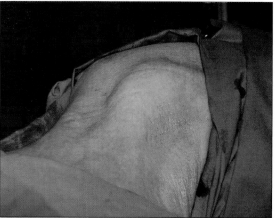

7.16 Aneurysm of the carotid artery. This is a rare cause of cerebrovascular symptoms. The aneurysm may contain clot and so act as a source of emboli to the brain. Therefore such aneurysms should usually be repaired. This patient had bilateral internal carotid aneurysms, which were repaired at separate procedures.

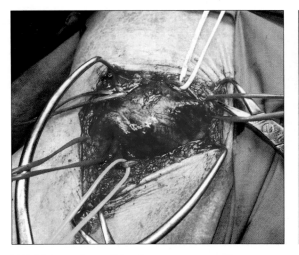

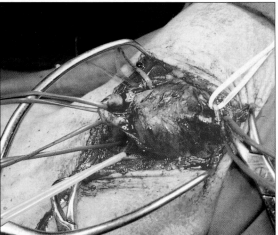

7.17 Internal carotid artery aneurysm. The aneurysm has been exposed and the common and internal carotid arteries are shown by red slings. The hypoglossal nerve is looped with a white sling and the vagus with a yellow sling. The external artery is looped with the blue sling.

7.18 Internal carotid artery aneurysm. Here the proximal internal carotid artery has been dissected out and the aneurysm is therefore wholly in the mid-internal carotid artery. It was possible to excise the aneurysm and perform an end-to-end anastomosis of the redundant and elongated, but normal calibre internal artery.

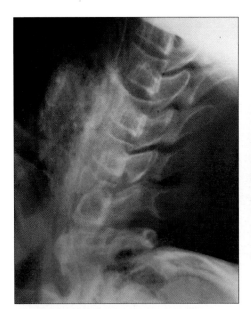

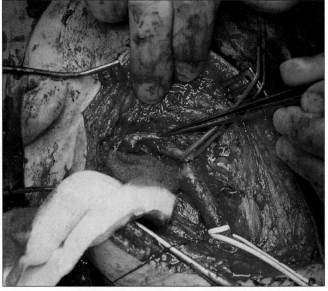

7.19 Chemodectoma. This angiogram shows the late view during carotid angiography, with the obvious tumour blush at the bifurcation. The bifurcation itself is generally markedly widened. Most cases present as asymptomatic lumps in the neck. Unfortunately, many are biopsied or explored without considering the possibility of a carotid body tumour as the diagnosis, rendering subsequent definitive surgery more hazardous.

7.20 Excision of carotid body tumour. Here, the tumour has been removed, effectively skeletonizing the carotid vessels. In most cases, as here, the external artery can be preserved. The hypoglossal nerve is identified at the upper border of the incision. Rarely, excision may be technically extremely difficult (often because of a previous effort at excision) and these cases are therefore best dealt with by a vascular surgeon familiar with shunting and carotid bypass techniques.

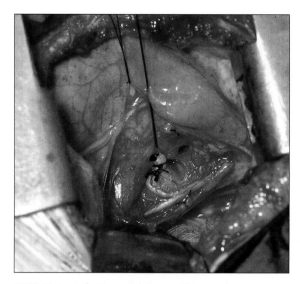

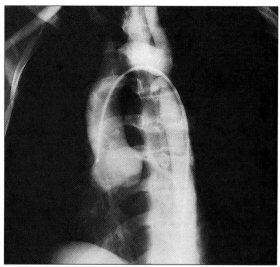

7.21 Patent ductus arteriosus. This vessel passes between the pulmonary artery and the arch or descending aorta. It is detected in infants and children with heart failure and a machinery-type murmur is heard over the pulmonary area. The ductus is shown with silk ties around it. The vagus nerve is visible, with the left recurrent laryngeal nerve curving around the lower margin of the ductus.

7.22 Coarctation of the aorta. Angiography shows a very tight stenosis of the descending aorta just beyond the left subclavian artery. Such patients can occasionally present in adult life with the lower body effectively supplied with blood flow provided by extensive arterial collateralization.

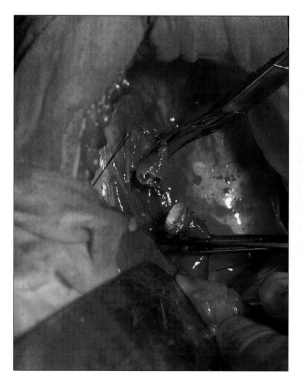

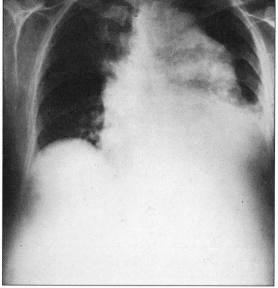

7.23 Coarctation of the aorta. The aorta has been divided at the level of a patent ductus. The artery held in the upper clamp has two lumens (the ductus and the proximal aorta) and there is a pinhole opening in the aorta proximal to the distal clamp.

7.24 Dissection of thoracic aorta. This classically presents with a tearing chest pain radiating into the back, and chest radiography will usually show a widened mediastinum, as here. Urgent arteriography and consideration of surgery are important because there is a high early mortality from rupture within the first 2 weeks (about 50%). Patients may present with a wide variety of symptoms including cerebrovascular symptoms, renal shutdown and leg ischaemia, depending upon which of the main aortic branches is involved in the process.

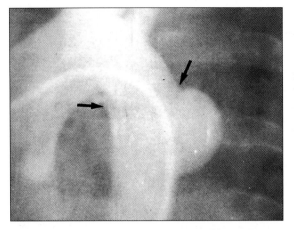

7.25 Traumatic aneurysm of the aorta. A young
man was involved in a road traffic accident and suffered a
deceleration injury to the thorax. This resulted in a partial
aortic tear, as seen here on angiography (arrows). Such
lesions should be repaired as soon as possible because they
are likely to rupture without warning.

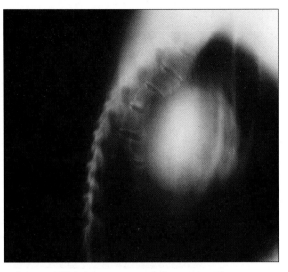

7.26 Syphilitic aneurysm of the aorta. This is now an
extremely rare phenomenon, but it was once the prinicipal
cause of thoracic aneurysms. Here, radiography shows
erosion of the thoracic vertebral bodies caused by a massive
syphilitic aneurysm, which is usually saccular.

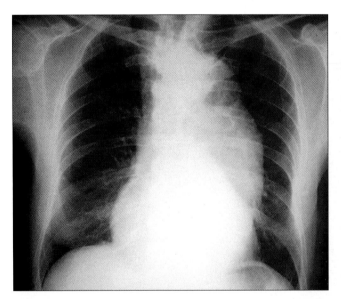

7.27 Descending thoracic aneurysm. Aneurysms of the
thoracic aorta may be isolated or form part of a larger
thoraco–abdominal aneurysm. Although not as common as abdominal
aortic aneurysms, they are just as likely to rupture and surgery should
always be considered if the patient is reasonably fit. Chest
radiography is the principal method of detecting such lesions because
most are asymptomatic unless they become extremely large. Definitive
diagnosis with magnetic resonance imaging (MRI) scans or
angiography is mandatory before considering surgery.

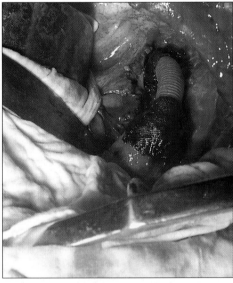

**7.28 Repair of a descending aortic
aneurysm.** This aneurysm arose distal to the left
subclavian artery and has been repaired with a
dacron graft, as shown. These operations may be
performed with a relatively low mortality and
morbidity provided the patient is reasonably fit. As
with carotid artery shunting, cardiac bypass using
femoro–femoral or atrio–femoral techniques or
shunts does not appear to have any great
advantage over the simpler 'clamp and graft'
approach.

8.

Aneurysms

An aneurysm is an abnormal dilatation of an artery, and may be classified into one of two types (**8.1**). The wall of a *true* aneurysm contains one or more of the histological layers of a normal artery wall. The wall of a *false* aneurysm contains none of the histological layers of a normal artery wall and results from trauma.

Causes of true and false aneurysms			
True		**False**	
Congenital	Marfan's syndrome	Injury	Penetrating (knife, gunshot)
	Ehlers–Danlos syndrome		Blunt (knee dislocation)
	Cerebral 'berry' aneurysm	Surgery	Graft dehiscence
Acquired	Atheromatous		Arteriotomy
	Mycotic		Lumbar disc operation
	Post-stenotic		
	Arteritides		
	Syphilitic		

8.1 Causes of true and false aneurysms.

The commonest form of aneurysm has been termed an 'atherosclerotic aneurysm', but this is probably not a valid description because although there is an association between aneurysmal disease and atheroma there is insufficient evidence to confirm a direct causal relationship.

Morphologically, aneurysms can be described as either fusiform (tapered at both ends) or saccular (sac-shaped) depending on whether there is diffuse or localized wall weakness, respectively.

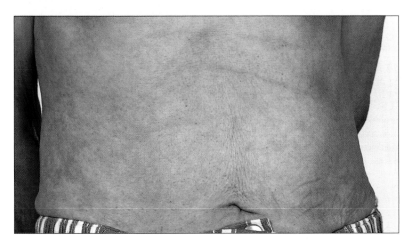

8.2 Abdominal aortic aneurysm. This is only palpable in 50% of cases. In these circumstances it is felt above the umbilicus as a painless mass with an expansile pulsation. It normally bulges to the left; this is because the aneurysm not only increases in transverse diameter, but also lengthens.

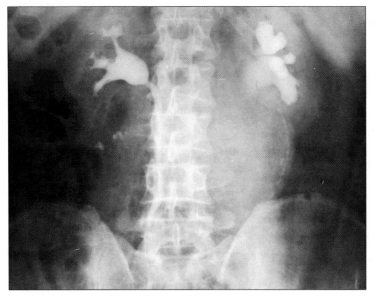

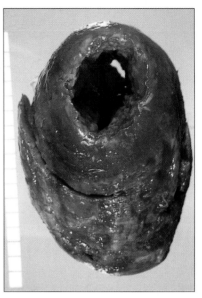

8.3 Calcification within the wall of the aorta. Plain postero–anterior or lateral radiographs will show calcification within the wall of the aorta and will suggest the diagnosis of abdominal aortic aneurysm in 80–90% of patients. As aneurysms tend to bulge to the left, the line of calcification is normally seen on the left side (the right side of the aneurysm overlying the spine). In this case the intravenous urogram also shows dilatation of the left renal pelvis, which may or may not be related to the aneurysm.

8.4 Mural laminated thrombus comprising most of the lumen of an aneurysm. It is generally the case that the true blood-containing lumen is only slightly larger than normal.

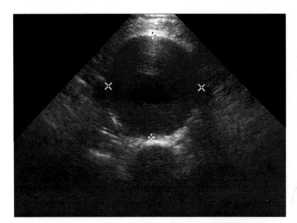

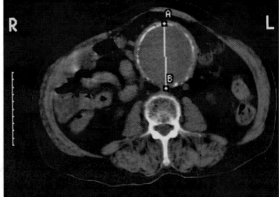

8.5 B-mode ultrasound of an aortic aneurysm. This is the routine method for investigating an aortic aneurysm. It reliably detects and sizes aneurysms, but is not the investigation of choice for determining the aneurysm's relationship to the renal arteries or diagnosing rupture. In the present scan the Xs mark the wall of the aneurysm and the majority of the lumen is occupied by mural thrombus, with the blood-containing lumen seen as the darker central section.

8.6 Computed tomography (CT) scanning of an aortic aneurysm. The most sensitive method for diagnosing an aortic aneurysm is CT scanning. (It also allows the diagnosis of an inflammatory aortic aneurysm by showing the thickened wall.)

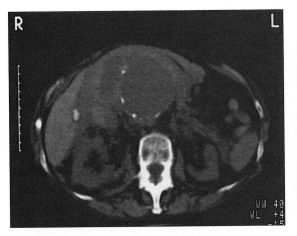

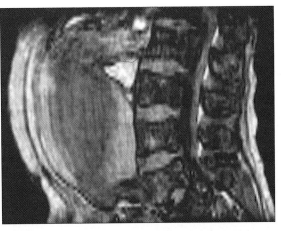

8.7 CT scan of a ruptured aortic aneurysm.
Blood/haematoma (darker material matching the intraluminal appearance) is shown on the right of a large aneurysm.

8.8 Magnetic resonance image of an aortic aneurysm (sagittal plane). This shows very fine detail of the aneurysm, but does not contribute significantly more than that provided by a CT scan.

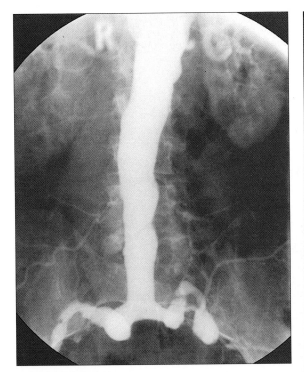

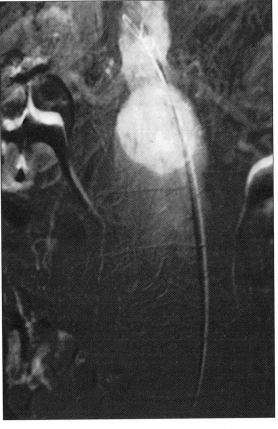

8.9 Angiography of an aortic aneurysm. This is generally restricted to the assessment of the aneurysm's anatomical relationship to the renal arteries and coincidental arterial disease affecting visceral or peripheral arteries. The presence of mural thrombus renders angiography inaccurate for the diagnosis and sizing of aortic aneurysms. In the present case there is an occlusion of the left external iliac artery and the aneurysm can be seen to extend above the level of the renal arteries.

8.10 Angiography of aortic aneurysms. This technique reveals that this abdominal aortic aneurysm originates below the renal vessels (as it does in 90% of cases).

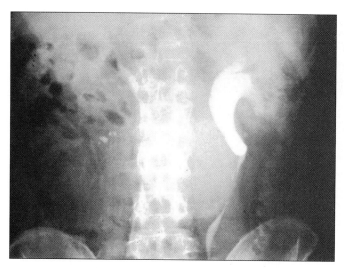

8.11 Very large aortic aneurysms. If very large, an aortic aneurysm may displace the ureter, though frank obstruction is rare unless there is also a degree of retroperitoneal fibrosis, which is associated with inflammatory aneurysms.

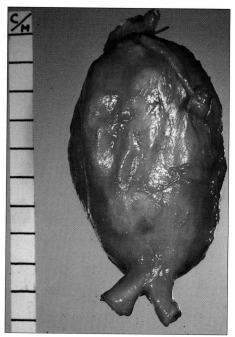

8.12 Aortic aneurysms may be restricted to the infrarenal aorta. This resected specimen shows an aortic aneurysm restricted to the infrarenal aorta. Alternatively they may also involve the iliac arteries. (Aneurysm resections are to all intents and purposes no longer performed.)

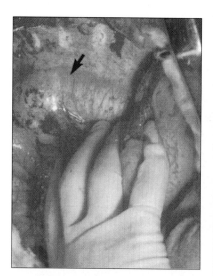

8.13 Thoracic aortic aneurysms may extend into the thoracic aorta and around to the aortic valve. This is relatively uncommon and is usually an incidental finding on a plain chest radiograph.

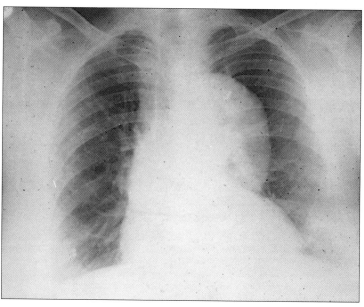

8.14 Chest radiograph of a thoracic aneurysm. This arch and descending parts of the aorta are widened on the chest radiograph.

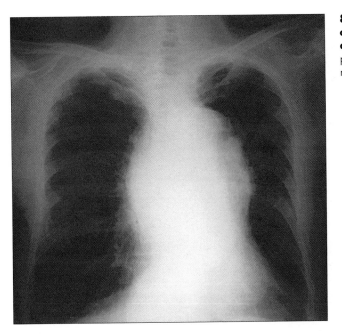

8.15 Syphilitic aneurysms used to be the commonest type of thoracic aortic aneurysm. Syphilitic aneurysms are the result of periarteritis and mesoarteritis, which weaken the media and give rise to dilatation.

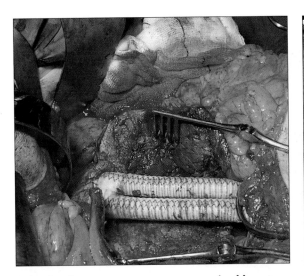

8.16 Aortic aneurysms are now repaired by an 'inlay' technique. The aneurysm is isolated and opened and a prosthetic graft is sutured to the proximal and distal margins inside the aneurysm sac.

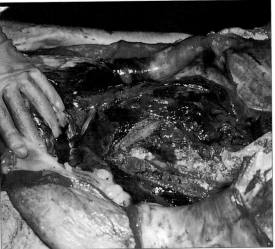

8.17 Rupture of an aortic aneurysm carries a very high mortality. Even with surgical repair the mortality may approach 95%. This is due to misdiagnosis of the cause of death, unsuitability for repair due to coexisting disease and finally a high operative mortality of 30–60%.

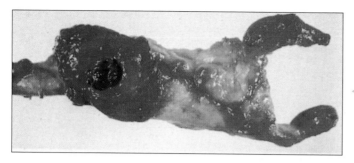

8.18 Aortoduodenal fistula. This may develop with rupture of the aorta into the gastrointestinal tract and presents as torrential haematemesis or rectal bleeding. Patients with an aortic reconstruction who then present with a major gastrointestinal haemorrhage should be assumed to have an aorto–duodenal fistula until proved otherwise at operation.

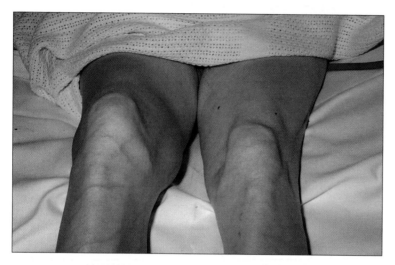

8.19 Popliteal artery aneurysm. These are not uncommon. They are commonly bilateral and can be associated with aneurysms at other sites (aorta and femoral). They tend to present with their complications: thrombosis leading to severe distal ischaemia; peripheral embolism (or 'trashing') with occlusion of small peripheral arteries; and least commonly, rupture. A generalized fullness above the right knee can be appreciated in this case.

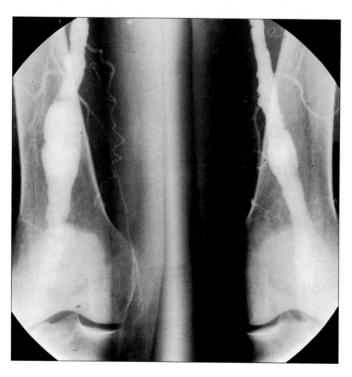

8.20 Angiogram of a popliteal aneurysm. A fusiform popliteal aneurysm is shown. Popliteal aneurysms like aortic aneurysms may be lined with mural thrombus. On thrombosis there is a sharp cut-off of contrast at the upper margins of the aneurysm with only poor outlining of more distal vessels.

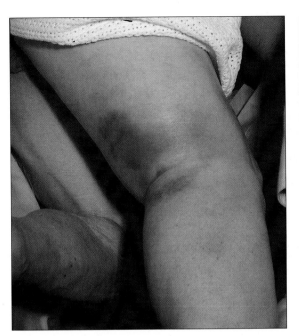

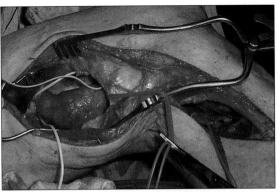

8.22 Operative exposure of a popliteal aneurysm. The aneurysm mainly involves the above-knee popliteal artery. The below-knee popliteal artery is seen to be of a normal calibre.

8.21 Rupture of a popliteal aneurysm. This is indicated by sudden and increasing pain associated with profuse bruising. There may or may not be distal ischaemia due to either compression or thrombosis.

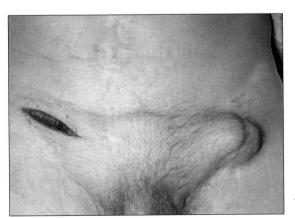

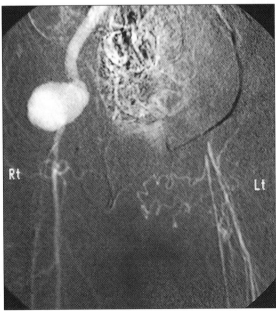

8.23 False femoral artery aneurysm. Usually this occurs at the anastomosis between the limb of an aortic bifurcation graft and the femoral arteries. In the example a large false aneurysm can be seen on the left, while on the right a leaking sinus has been explored.

8.24 Intravenous digital subtraction angiogram (i.v. DSA) of an anastomotic aneurysm at the femoral anastomosis of an aortic bifurcated graft. A large false aneurysm, which required a short interposition graft to bridge the gap, is shown.

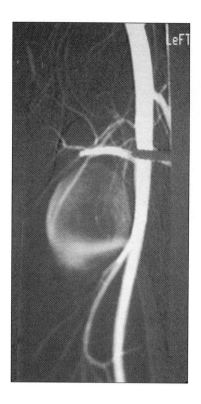

8.25 False aneurysms may also be iatrogenic due to other mechanisms. The commonest mechanism is probably following arterial catherization for peripheral or cardiac angiographic procedures. The example shown followed orthopaedic repair of a femoral head fracture in a young motorcyclist. The aneurysm is arising from the profunda femoris artery.

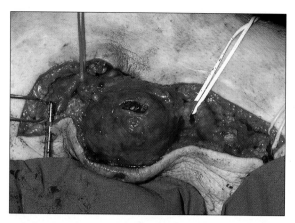

8.26 Vein graft aneurysms are very uncommon. Nevertheless they are subject to the same complications as lower limb arterial aneurysms and should be treated identically by operative repair.

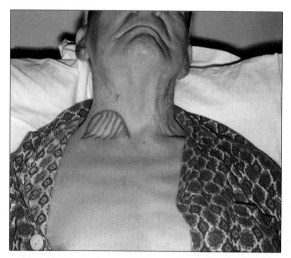

8.27 Subclavian aneurysm. This is outlined in the left supraclavicular fossa. It is a very rare aneurysm and may be intimately involved with the brachial plexus.

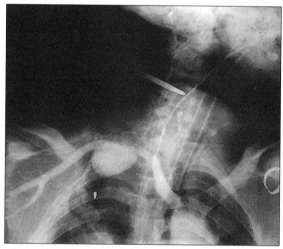

8.28 Angiogram of subclavian aneurysm. A saccular aneurysm overlying the apex of the right lung is demonstrated.

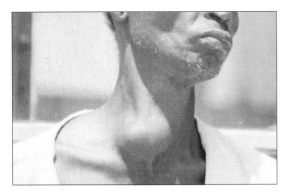

8.29 Syphilitic subclavian aneurysm. Now virtually never seen in developed countries, this example is arising from the first part of the subclavian artery.

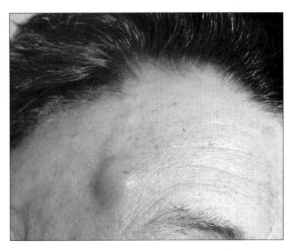

8.30 Temporal artery aneurysm. This is usually due to blunt trauma following a fall and is therefore a false aneurysm. Intervention is only warranted if the aneurysm is expanding or causing distress. In this case the aneurysm was mycotic in origin.

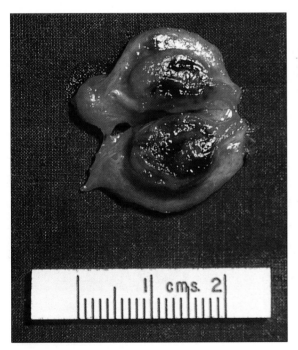

8.31 Mycotic aneurysm. The aneurysm shown here can be seen to be due to localized weakening of the arterial wall by infection, resulting in a false aneurysm.

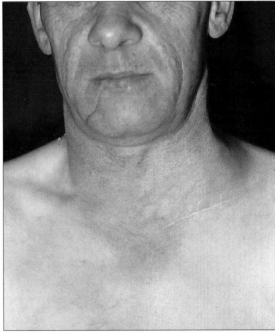

8.32 Mycotic aneurysm of the subclavian artery. The same patient as in **8.31** returned a year later with a mycotic aneurysm of the left subclavian artery. This is a very rare site for the development of this type of aneurysm.

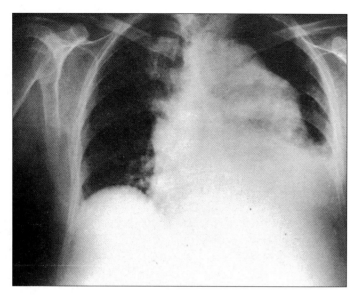

8.33 Dissecting aneurysm is a minor misnomer. Aneurysms do not dissect because the dilating process tends to seal the necessary layers together. Nevertheless a dissecting aneurysm is still an aneurysm, but one due to dissection. The patient classically presents with tearing back pain, shock and dyspnoea. A plain chest radiograph reveals a broadened mediastinum and fluid (blood) collection in the left pleural space.

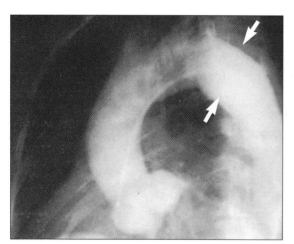

8.34 Angiogram of a dissecting aneurysm. This shows the double lumen of the false and true lumen (arrows). The origin/entry into the false lumen may begin at the aortic valve, in the ascending aorta or just distal to the origin of the left subclavian artery.

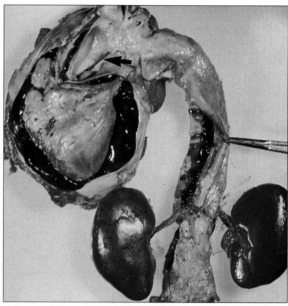

8.35 Type 1 dissecting aneurysm. This begins about 2 cm distal to the aortic valve (arrowed) and proceeds down the abdominal aorta and back into the peritoneal sac.

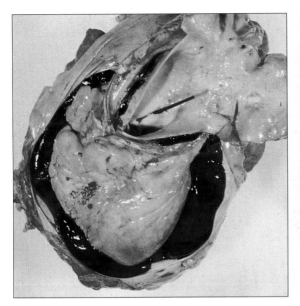

8.36 Aortic wall tear. This is more easily shown in a closer view. The causes of death were cardiac tamponade and aortic valve failure.

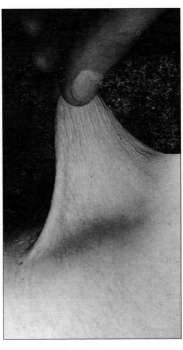

8.37 Ehlers–Danlos syndrome. This is a connective tissue disorder resulting in a loss of elasticity of the tissues, demonstrated here in the skin. Both this and Marfan's syndrome are associated with aneurysms due to dissection.

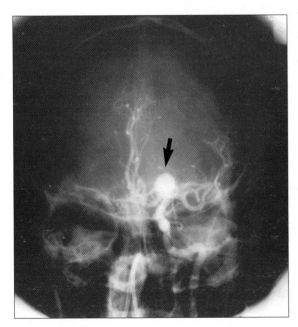

8.38 Berry aneurysm of the left internal carotid bifurcation. This is seen on a conventional cerebral angiogram. The aneurysm is caused by a congenital weakness within the wall of the artery, usually at a point of bifurcation.

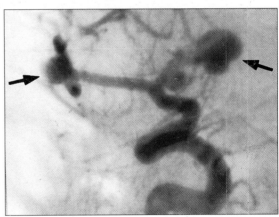

8.39 Berry aneurysms of the circle of Willis. These are shown (arrows) on an intra-arterial digital subtraction angiogram. The carotid siphon is clearly seen leading to the circle of Willis.

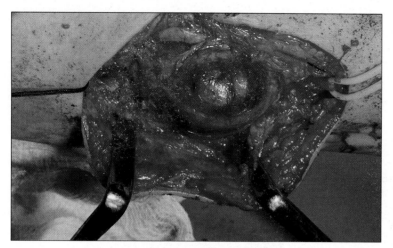

8.40 Radial artery aneurysm. This was the presumptive diagnosis. The swelling exhibited an expansile pulsation in a common site of radial artery injury.

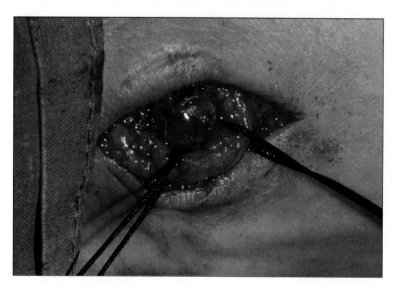

8.41 Radial artery overlying a ganglion. In this case of suspected radial artery aneurysm the actual diagnosis, as shown by this operative picture, was of the radial artery being displaced superficially by a deep-placed ganglion. The swelling would not move from side to side and did not collapse on pressure. Prominent arterial pulsation due to a tortuous vessel resulting from vessel lengthening can also be confused with an aneurysm, the classical sites being the carotid artery or aorta.

9.

Vasospasm

Man is a tropical creature, better suited to losing heat than retaining it. His neutral environmental temperature when naked and at rest is 28°C. After a fall of only 8°C in environmental temperature, his metabolic rate must double or his body temperature will fall.

Man's response to cold, the putting on of clothes, enables him to survive in temperate areas. However, some people respond abnormally to cold. The best recognized of these cold-related vascular disorders is Raynaud's phenomenon.

RAYNAUD'S PHENOMENON

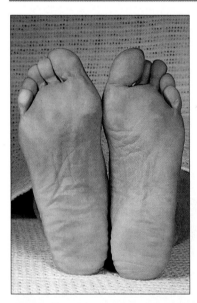

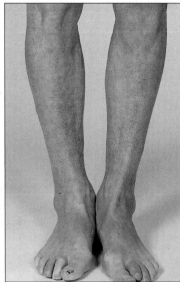

9.1 Raynaud's phenomenon. This condition affects 5–10% of the population and is nine times more common in women than in men. It is subdivided into Raynaud's syndrome in which there is an associated disorder and Raynaud's disease where there is not. It is classically manifest by pallor, reflecting vasospasm in the digital vessels, and although usually reported in the hands, it may also affect the feet, as seen here. The dorsa of both the great toes are blanched, as are some of the other toes. On the plantar surface of the foot the vasospasm extends over the metatarsal heads.

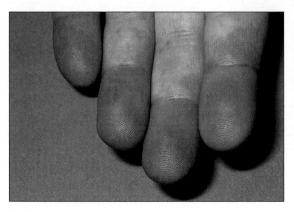

9.2 Cyanosis. Intermittent blanching is the cardinal diagnostic feature for Raynaud's phenomenon. This is often followed by cyanosis as seen here, where there is deoxygenation of the blood trapped in the vasospastic vessels.

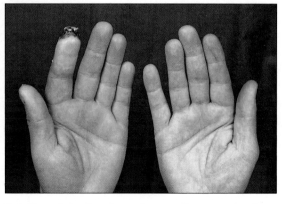

9.3 The triphasic colour change. This is completed during the reactive hyperaemic phase of Raynaud's phenomenon when there is a return of blood flow to the extremity. The reactive hyperaemia may be accompanied by the symptom of rewarming paraesthesia.

Immunological disorders	Occupational
Systemic sclerosis	Vibration white-finger disease
Mixed connective tissue disease	Cold injury
Dermatomyositis/polymyositis	Vinyl-chloride workers
Systemic lupus erythematosus	**Drugs**
Rheumatoid arthritis	
Cold agglutinins	Unselective beta blockers
Obstructive arterial disease	Ergot and other antimigraine drugs
	Cytotoxic agents
Atherosclerosis including Buerger's disease	**Miscellaneous**
Thoracic outlet syndromes	Idiopathic Raynaud's disease
Emboli	Hypothyroidism
	? Neoplasm

9.4 Associated disorders.
Although primary Raynaud's disease is the most common form of the disorder, approximately 50% of patients with symptoms severe enough for hospital referral have an underlying cause. This table shows the main conditions and causative factors associated with Raynaud's phenomenon.

CONNECTIVE TISSUE DISEASE

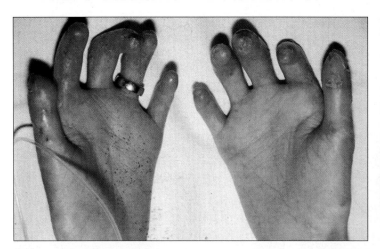

9.5 Connective tissue disease. The most frequently seen secondary form of Raynaud's phenomenon is that associated with the connective tissue disorders. Systemic sclerosis is the most common diagnosis, and in the later stages, sclerodactyly (tightening of the skin of the fingers) contributes significantly to the digital ischaemia, as seen here.

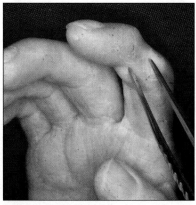

9.6 Systemic sclerosis. This may be diffuse if there is widespread or limited organ involvement. Limited systemic sclerosis, formerly called the CREST syndrome (Calcinosis, Raynaud's, oEsophagitis, Sclerodactyly, Telangiectasia), may be complicated by calcinosis. These are subcutaneous deposits of small calcium granules, which are very irritant.

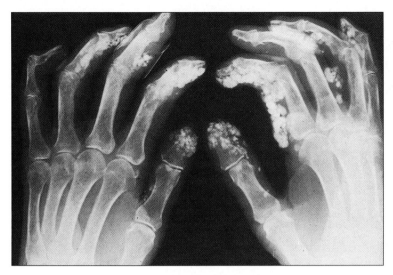

9.7 Calcinosis. The granules work their way to the surface where they ulcerate through the skin. Digital ulceration and infection follow. This radiograph clearly shows the subcutaneous calcium deposits.

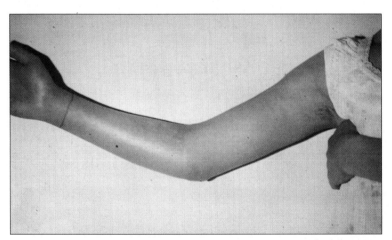

9.8 Scleroderma means 'hard skin'. Diffuse systemic sclerosis progresses to tightened and thickened skin. This is termed 'sclerodactyly' in the fingers and 'scleroderma' on the limbs and trunk.

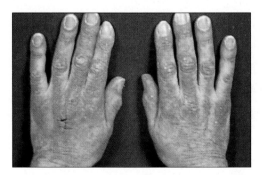

9.9 Polymyositis and dermatomyositis. These conditions are closely related and the pathology is one of inflammation of the muscles and skin. Patients may have difficulty lifting their arms and getting up and down the stairs. Involvement of the skin gives rise to a heliotrope rash on the eyelids. In the hands, as seen here, Goddrons' patches may be found. These are scaly erythematous lesions over the dorsa of the hands.

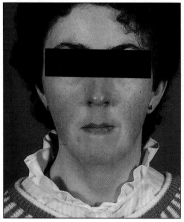

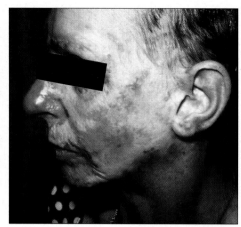

9.11 Systemic lupus erythematosus. This condition is characterized by photosensitivity of exposed areas. The extent of the inflammation can be such that scarring occurs, as is seen here. Another feature of systemic lupus erythematosus is alopecia.

9.10 Systemic lupus erythematosus. Skin involvement is the commonest presenting feature in systemic lupus erythematosus. This may manifest as the blanching of Raynaud's syndrome, periungual infarcts, palpable purpura or livedo reticularis. Classically an erythematous sun-sensitive rash appears over the malar region of the face and over the bridge of the nose—the well-described butterfly rash, which is seen here.

Clinical features
Isolated features of connective tissue disease
Digital ulceration
Assymetry of vasospasm
Return chilblains
Attacks all year round
Older age of onset of Raynaud's
Abnormal nailfold vessels
Tortuosity
Dilatation
Vessel 'drop out'
Positive immunological tests
Antinuclear antibody
Rheumatoid factor
Extractable nuclear antigens
e.g. Scleroderma 70
Anticentromere
Ro/La

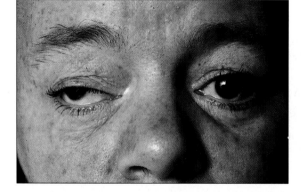

9.12 Systemic lupus erythematosus. Cerebral vessel involvement in the form of a vasculitis can also be a feature of systemic lupus erythematosus. This illustration shows the demonstration of a third nerve palsy in a patient with this disorder.

9.13 Differentiating primary and secondary Raynaud's phenomenon. This can be of critical importance to the patient in terms of follow-up, treatment and prognosis. A number of clinical and laboratory features that provide the clinician with good diagnostic pointers can be evaluated.

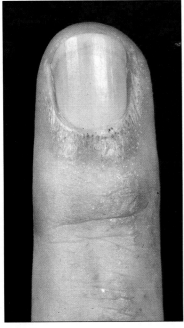

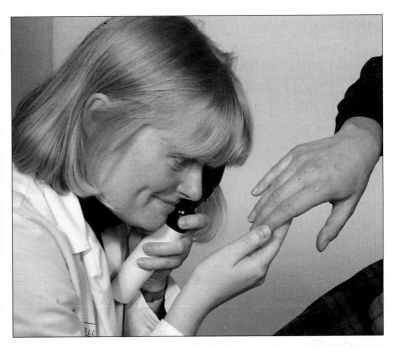

9.14 Abnormal nailfold vessels. In addition to the clinical and laboratory features shown above, abnormalities of the nailfold vasculature seen on microscopic examination can occur. In connective tissue disease the nailfold vessels become dilated and tortuous and may even become occluded (capillary dropout) in severe cases. These abnormalities can be clearly seen here with the naked eye as small red lines drawing back from the nail cuticle.

9.15 Microscopy. High-powered microscopy provides good views of abnormal vessels early in the progression of connective tissue disease, but a lower-powered instrument can still be useful. If an ophthalmoscope at highest magnification, is held a few millimetres above the nailfold area, early abnormalities of vessels can be detected as small pink thread lines.

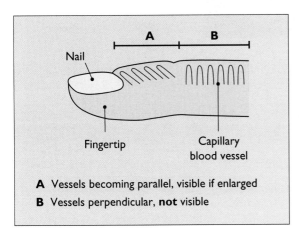

A Vessels becoming parallel, visible if enlarged
B Vessels perpendicular, **not** visible

9.16 Abnormal nailfold vessels. The nailfold area is the best place for study because developmentally the vessels fold over towards the nail, becoming parallel to the skin surface. When these are combined with abnormalities of rheumatoid arthritis latex test, antinuclear antibody or extractable nuclear antigen titres, there is a 90% likelihood of subsequent development of connective tissue disease. Abnormal nailfold vessels can also be seen in diabetes mellitus and after trauma, such as that induced by nailfold biting.

OCCUPATIONAL RAYNAUD'S PHENOMENON

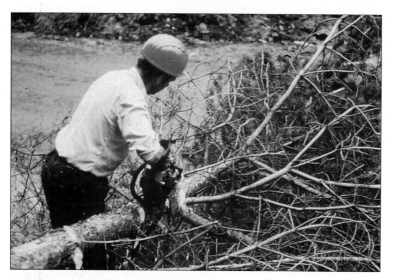

9.17 Vibration exposure.
Vibration exposure is the commonest cause of Raynaud's phenomenon in men. Classically it is associated with forestry workers in the context of tree felling, for which power chain saws, as shown here, were commonly used. Modern equipment is now specifically designed to produce vibration levels outside the frequency bands that induce vibration white finger disease (*see* **9.19**).

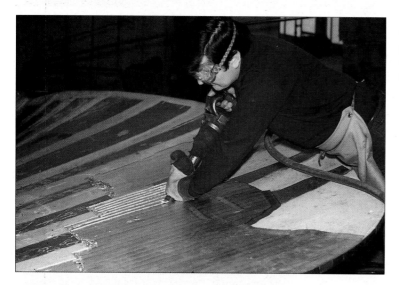

9.18 Other vibratory machines.
These can also cause problems and include grinders, buffs and drills. In women, industrial polishers and sewing machines have been implicated.

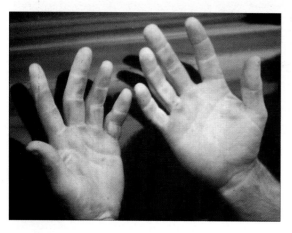

9.19 Vibration white finger disease. Blanching of the digits, as seen here, occurs in 20–80% of workers exposed to vibration after a variable latent period. This may be associated with vibration-induced peripheral nerve damage, which manifests initially as a constant paraesthesia and subsequently as numbness. Vibration also injures the joints and for this reason the condition is also called hand/arm vibration syndrome. Diagnosis is by the exclusion of other secondary forms of Raynaud's syndrome combined with a history of vibration exposure. It is now a recognized industrial disease attracting financial compensation if employers are found negligent in protecting their staff from vibration effects.

Stage	Condition of digits	Work and social interference
0	No blanching of digits	No complaints
OT	Intermittent tingling	No interference with activities
ON	Intermittent numbness	No interference with activities
1	Blanching of one or more fingertips with or without tingling and numbness	No interference with activities
2	Blanching of one or more fingers with numbness; usually confined to winter	Slight interference with home and social activities; no interference at work
3	Extensive blanching; frequent episodes during the summer as well as winter	Definite interference at work, at home and with social activities; restriction of hobbies
4	Extensive blanching of most fingers; frequent episodes summer and winter	Occupation changed to avoid further vibration exposure because of severity of signs and symptoms

9.20 Severity grading. This can be carried out in vibration white finger disease using a number of established scales. These include clinical assessment scales such as the Taylor–Pelmear Scale illustrated here.

COLD INJURY

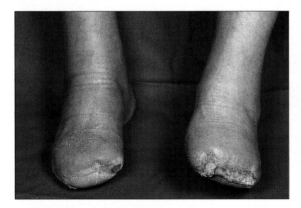

9.21 Cold-induced damage. This occurs as a result of vasoconstriction (which decreases blood flow), endothelial damage (which is prothrombotic), crystallization of blood constituents and direct tissue freezing. It can occur during the course of the patient's occupation, as seen here. This soldier developed 'trench foot' and lost his toes after exposure to cold in the trenches of World War I.

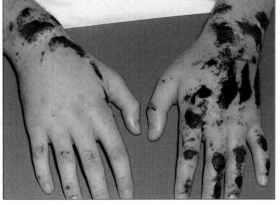

9.22 Frostbite. This can be produced by outdoor recreational sports when the vasculature in the tissues has been frozen by a dry cold. This patient is a mountaineer. A few weeks later, with conservative management, an excellent recovery was made. Loss of digits can occur in more extreme cases.

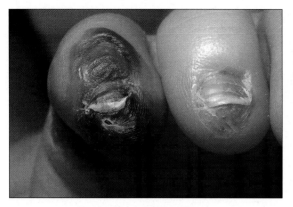

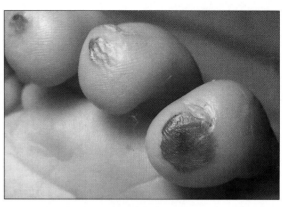

9.23 Temperature perception. As this is altered in the very young and old, these groups are vulnerable to hypothermia and cold injury. The toes in this child's foot were exposed to cold due to defective socks, the ends of which were worn off, exposing the tips of the toes to cold.

9.24 Cold injury to toes. The toes of the other foot were similarly, but less severely, affected by the cold.

OBSTRUCTIVE ARTERIAL DISEASE

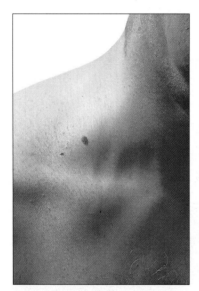

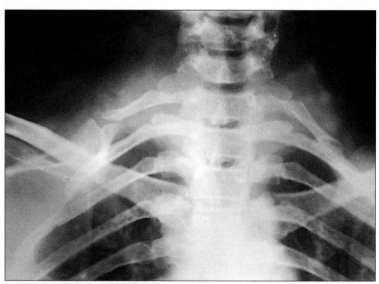

9.25 Attacks of unilateral Raynaud's phenomenon. These often suggest an underlying cause, which include thoracic outlet syndromes such as the presence of a cervical rib, as seen here, where there is a prominence within the right supraclavicular fossa. Although symptoms may be unilateral, cervical ribs are often found on both sides.

9.26 Bilateral cervical ribs. Plane radiograph of the neck showing bilateral cervical ribs. The one on the left side is more prominent than that on the right.

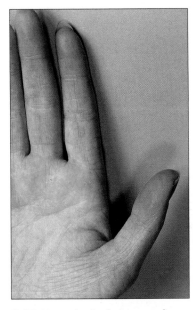

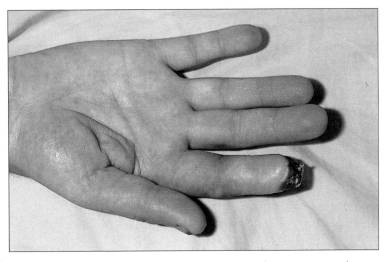

9.28 Vascular changes. These can be more serious than mere Raynaud's phenomenon. In this illustration, digital gangrene has resulted due to pressure on the vessel from the rib with possible distal embolization.

9.27 Neurological signs and symptoms. A cervical rib may cause neurological signs and symptoms indicative of brachial plexus involvement. The patient may complain of paraesthesia and there may be signs of small muscle wasting, in addition to the ischaemia, as seen here. The index finger felt cold and a slight bluish tinge was seen in the pulp of the finger.

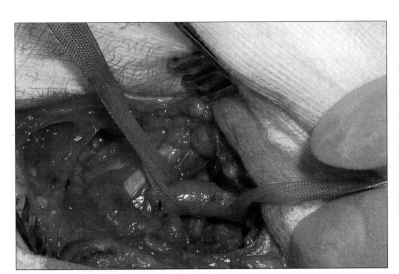

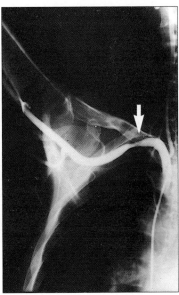

9.29 Cervical rib. Surgical removal of the cervical rib may be required in severely affected patients. The rib can be seen here under the elevated subclavian artery. Residual damage may, however, persist postoperatively.

9.30 The subclavian artery. This artery may also be narrowed as a result of thoracic outlet compression (arrow) due to other causes. In this case it was thought to be due to the pressure of the muscles as the arm was hyperabducted.

ATHEROSCLEROSIS

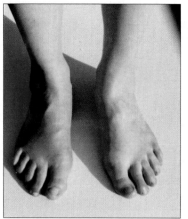
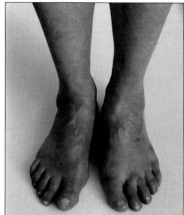

9.31 Raynaud's phenomenon. Raynaud's phenomenon with an onset in someone over 60 years of age is likely to be related to generalized atherosclerotic Raynaud's phenomenon particularly occurs in diabetics. Although blanching may be the primary feature, the reactive hyperaemia is often the most troublesome symptom. The patient's main complaint is of hot/burning extremities (i.e. erythromelalgia).

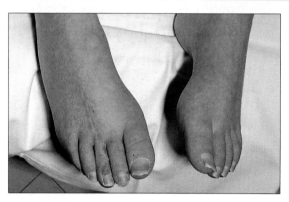

9.32 Erythromelalgia. This can be troublesome, particularly when the vasospasm affects the feet. It can give rise to bizarre behavioural patterns such as sleeping with the feet sticking out of the window or immersed in buckets of ice. This patient had severe erythromelalgia, which made sleep at night impossible. She subsequently developed trophic changes in her toes, as seen here, due to repeated immersion in iced water.

PHARMACOLOGICALLY INDUCED VASOSPASM

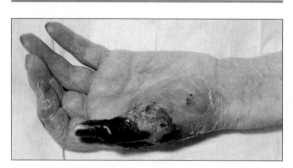

9.33 Drugs. A number of commonly used drugs can cause a varying degree of vasospasm. These include beta blockers, which are commonly prescribed for associated cardiovascular symptoms such as angina. Migraine is also associated with Raynaud's phenomenon and some migraine treatments may cause vasoconstriction. The most severe form of chemically induced vasospasm can be seen in drug addicts who either deliberately or inadvertently inject irritant drugs into their arteries. This man was an addict who unfortunately injected his 'fix' into the brachial artery.

REFLEX SYMPATHETIC DYSTROPHY

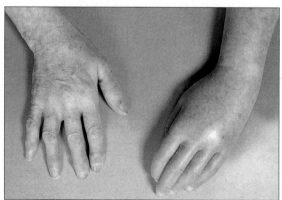

9.34 Reflex sympathetic dystrophy. Injury to the neck, shoulder or limb may result in chronic vasoconstriction in which the extremities are bluish and cold. There may be associated neurological signs and subsequent development of osteoporosis. This condition is painful and is often called causalgia. Here the patient's left hand is swollen and the skin shiny, and the burning pain experienced is characteristic.

ACROCYANOSIS

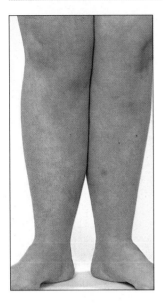

9.35 Acrocyanosis. The aetiology of acrocyanosis is also vasospastic. The site of the spasm, however, is in the postcapillary venules; the primary manifestation is therefore cyanosis of the area secondary to deoxygenation of the blood trapped in the capillaries. This is a benign condition, but the cyanosis may concern the patient, who should be reassured. It is fairly refractory to drug treatment. The affected limb may be cold, and as here, the cyanosis may have a reticular pattern.

MANAGEMENT

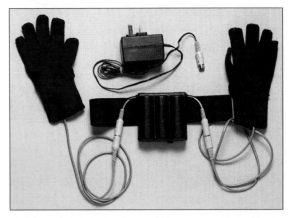

9.36 Management of Raynaud's phenomenon. This depends on the correct diagnosis of any underlying condition. If none can be found then primary Raynaud's disease may be diagnosed. This condition is often self-limiting and not usually severe enough to warrant drug treatment. Electrically heated gloves, which obtain their power from rechargeable batteries worn round the waist, may be ideal for young girls or women with Raynaud's disease.

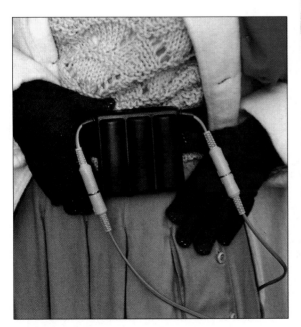

9.37 Electric gloves. A battery belt is provided. The wires from the battery go down the sleeve to the glove and are hidden by the outdoor clothing. The battery is fairly heavy, however, and frail elderly patients with Raynaud's phenomenon are unlikely to be able to use this form of treatment.

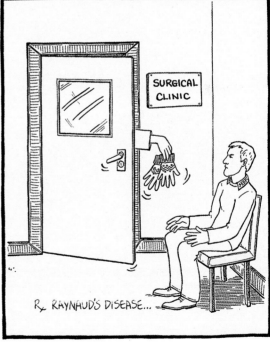

9.38 Drug treatment. Until recently, drug treatment for Raynaud's phenomenon had been poorly evaluated. In the past, many patients were merely told to stay indoors, keep warm and wear gloves. More recently, good scientific clinical trials have made it clear that some treatments can benefit these patients.

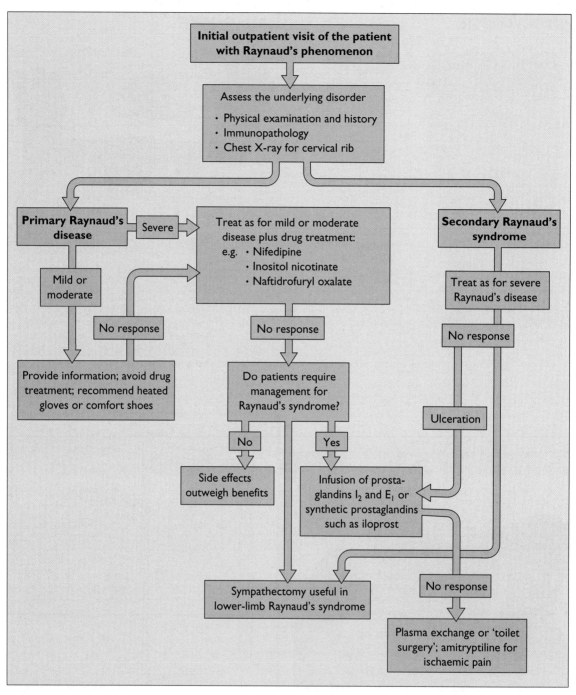

9.39 Drug treatment. This may be required for patients with severe primary Raynaud's disease and also for those with secondary Raynaud's syndrome. A flow chart, such as the one shown here, can usually be followed.

10.

Vasculitides

The vasculitides are all characterized by inflammation within the blood vessel wall, with impairment of blood flow and possibly damage to vessel integrity. The vasculitic process may involve only one or many blood vessels and therefore organ systems. In general, the clinical features result from ischaemia to the tissues supplied by the damaged vessels and are often accompanied by the systemic features of fever, weight loss and anorexia, which result from widespread inflammation. These conditions produce a range of symptoms from a mild obliterative disorder to necrotizing vasculitis.

Type of vasculitis	Aorta and its branches	Large and medium-sized arteries	Medium-sized muscular arteries	Small muscular arteries	Arterioles, capillaries and venules
Takayasu's arteritis	●				
Buerger's disease (thromboangiitis obliterans)	●	●			
Giant cell arteritis (temporal arteritis)	●	●			
Polyarteritis nodosa		●	●		
Wegener's granulomatosis			●	●	
Connective tissue diseases				●	●
Rheumatoid vasculitis				●	●
Cutaneous vasculitis (leucocytoclastic vasculitis)					●

10.1 Size of vessel. Vessels of predominantly one or many types may be affected and this table shows some of the common vasculitides stratified by the size of vessel most commonly involved.

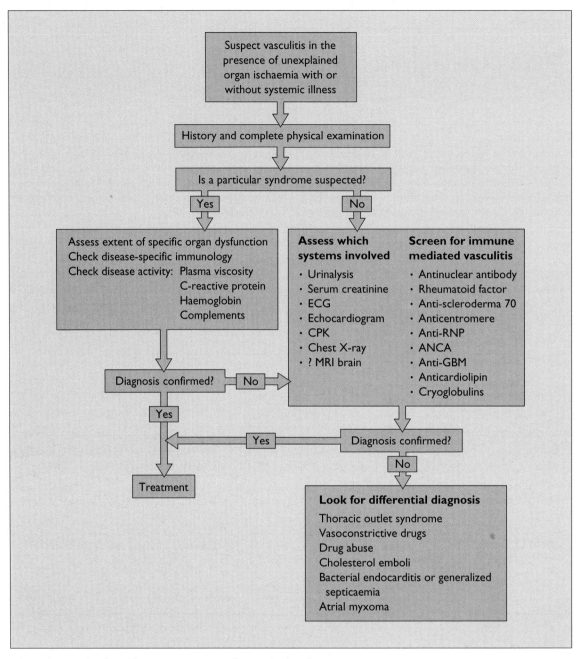

10.2 Diagnostic algorithm. Diagnosing specific vasculitides often requires specialist intervention. Nevertheless, the algorithm shown here outlines a possible initial investigation strategy that may be helpful. ANCA = antineutrophil cytoplasmic antibody; CPK = creatinine phosphokinase; GBM = glomerular basement membrane.

TAKAYASU'S ARTERITIS

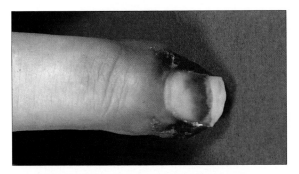

10.3 Takayasu's arteritis. This is a chronic inflammatory disorder of unknown aetiology that primarily affects the aorta and its major branches, producing symptoms in the upper limb as seen here. It most commonly occurs in women under 40 years of age, but older women and men may also be affected. This 28-year-old woman also required a below-knee amputation of the left leg. The right leg is also affected.

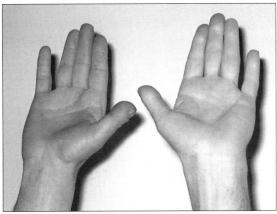

10.4 Upper limb claudication. This is common and is associated with reduced or absent upper limb pulses. Pallor of the affected arm is clearly seen in this illustration.

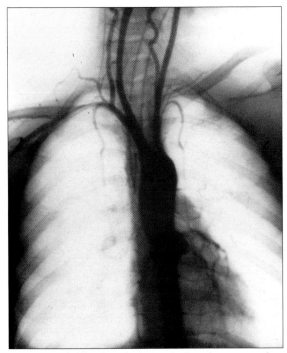

10.5 Arterial bruits. These may be heard over carotid, abdominal and subclavian vessels. The angiogram shows narrowing of the subclavian arteries, and this appearance in a young woman is typical of the aortic arch syndrome of Takayasu's disease. The clinical features may include the systemic symptoms of fever, night sweats and fatigue. Immunosuppressive treatment is often required.

BUERGER'S DISEASE

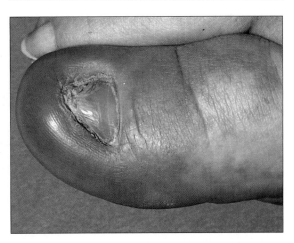

10.6 Buerger's disease (thromboangiitis obliterans). This condition is characterized by the occurrence of segmental thrombotic occlusions of the small- and medium-sized arteries, usually of the distal lower extremities, as seen here, but also involving the upper limb. This 42-year-old man had easily palpable femoral and popliteal pulses.

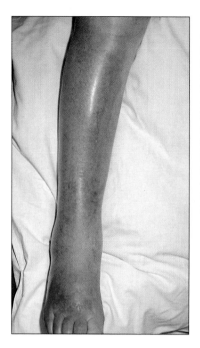

10.7 Buerger's disease. Usually this condition occurs in young male smokers, but is now occurring more frequently in women. It is also associated with both Raynaud's syndrome and superficial migratory thrombophlebitis. This latter condition can be clearly seen here in this 46-year-old man who smoked 40 cigarettes a day.

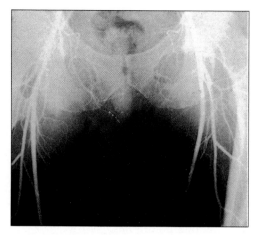

10.8 Buerger's disease. The condition appears clinically and pathologically distinct from both atherosclerosis and various forms of immune-mediated vasculitis. On this angiogram, the lower part of the superficial femoral arteries show a smooth narrowing in a tapering fashion. This emphasizes the link between Buerger's disease and atherosclerosis, which nearly always coexist. Histology of the resected toes confirmed the presence of vasculitis.

GIANT CELL ARTERITIS

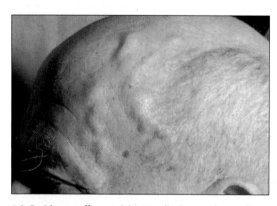

10.9 Giant cell arteritis. Usually this condition affects the elderly and is a vasculitis of unknown aetiology. It is also known as temporal arteritis, cranial arteritis or granulomatous arteritis. The clinical symptoms relate to the arteries involved and include headache, which may be accompanied by a prominent temporal artery, as seen here. Later, the temporal artery pulse may disappear as the vessel occludes.

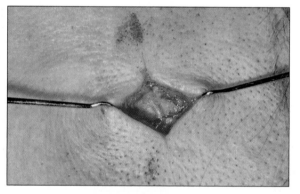

10.10 Temporal artery biopsy. A diagnosis of giant cell arteritis can be confirmed by temporal artery biopsy. Multinuclear giant cells are diagnostic, but remember that 'skip lesions' occur and a negative biopsy does not exclude the diagnosis. Jaw claudication, loss of vision and polymyalgia rheumatica are common features, and early recognition and treatment with steroids can prevent blindness and other complications due to occlusion or rupture of the involved arteries. The erythrocyte sedimentation rate or plasma viscosity is usually markedly elevated, but can be normal in 2% of patients.

POLYARTERITIS NODOSA

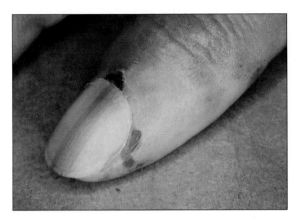

10.11 Polyarteritis nodosa. This condition is characterized by inflammation of small- and medium-sized arteries involving the skin, kidney, nerves, gut and muscle. Skin manifestations include nailfold infarcts, as seen here, palpable purpura, and livedo reticularis.

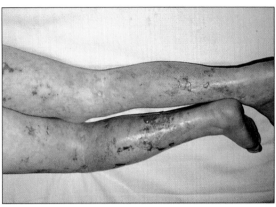

10.12 Skin infarction. This can result in tissue death and gangrene, as seen here.

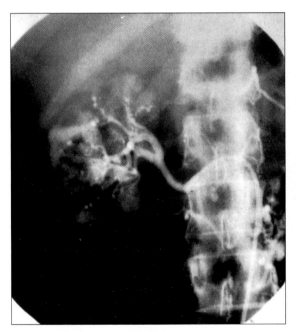

10.13 Polyarteritis nodosa. Virtually any organ can be affected and therefore the disease may present in a variety of ways. Damage to the vessel wall can result in aneurysm formation, as demonstrated here on this renal arteriogram.

CONNECTIVE TISSUE DISEASES

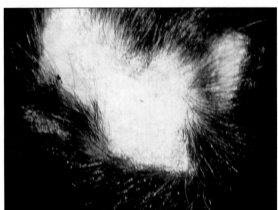

10.14 Systemic lupus erythematosus (SLE). This is an inflammatory multisystem disease with diverse clinical and laboratory manifestations. It often presents with a butterfly skin rash, as shown in **9.10**, or arthralgia. The clinical features reflect inflammation in various organs (e.g. brain, kidney), and this inflammation can also affect the blood vessels—SLE vasculitis. Splinter infarcts may be accompanied by other signs of skin ischaemia, as shown here in this patient with SLE and alopecia.

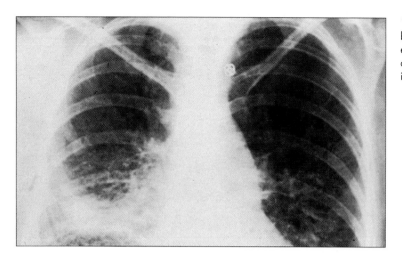

10.15 Pneumonitis. This may also be a feature of systemic lupus erythematosus when inflammation occurs in the lung. It is treated with immunosuppressive therapy.

RHEUMATOID ARTHRITIS

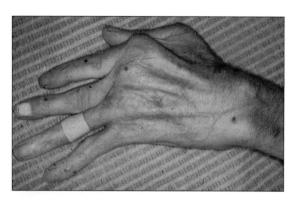

10.16 Rheumatoid arthritis. This reasonably common arthritis may be associated with vasculitis. Occlusion of small vessels produces skin infarcts, which are seen here in conjunction with the classic joint changes in the hand, including ulnar deviation and subluxation of the metacarpophalangeal joints.

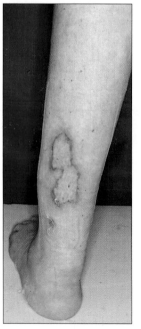

10.17 Vasculitic ulceration. This may be a feature in rheumatoid arthritis and can be misdiagnosed unless the diagnosis of rheumatoid arthritis is actively considered. This patient had a leg ulcer for 9 years. It was thought to be varicose in origin, but no varicose veins were present. The patient had rheumatoid arthritis, and biopsy established the ulcer to be vasculitic.

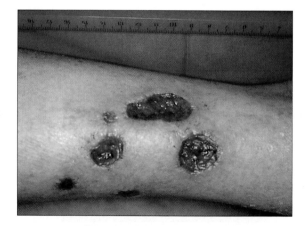

10.18 Vasculitic ulcers. These are often described as having a 'punched out' appearance. Here the well-demarcated margins are clearly seen, with normal skin surrounding the ulcerated area. Often, inflammation within and around the ulcer is also a feature of vasculitic ulcers. Purely ischaemic ulcers occurring in an ischaemic limb do not have sufficient local blood flow to mount an inflammatory response.

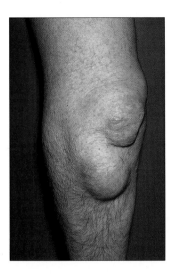

10.19 Rheumatoid nodules. These are areas of vasculitis. They are found over bony prominences and along tendon sheaths. They should always be looked for in cases of unexplained lower limb ulceration. In this illustration rheumatoid nodules are clearly demonstrated over the extensor surface of the elbow.

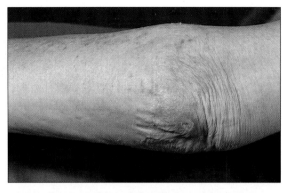

10.20 Rheumatoid nodules. These nodules may ulcerate due to ischaemia secondary to vessel inflammation. The ulcers heal poorly and are liable to become a source of infection in the rheumatoid patient.

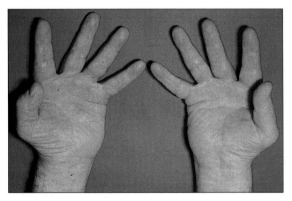

10.21 Clinical features of rheumatoid arthritis. These are easy to detect when the patient has severe disease and obvious deformities. Less easy to diagnose is the patient illustrated here, who has mild ulnar deviation and deformity affecting the right metacarpophalangeal thumb joint.

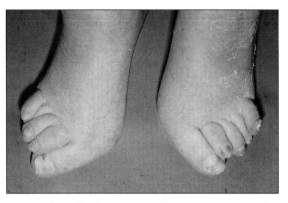

10.22 Ulnar deviation. This refers to the subluxation of the metacarpophalangeal joints and subsequent ulnar deviation of the fingers. For ease of reference, this term is also applied to the lateral deviation of the toes due to metatarsal subluxation, as seen in this slide.

CUTANEOUS VASCULITIS

Drugs	Immunological disorders	Infections
Antibiotics	Connective tissue disease	Upper respiratory tract viruses
Penicillins	Cryoglobulinaemia	Streptococcus with or without bacterial endocarditis
Sulphonamides	Allergic granulomatosis (Churg–Strauss syndrome)	
Diuretics		Hepatitis B infection
Nonsteroidal anti-inflammatories	Behcet's disease	
Anticonvulsants		

10.23 Cutaneous vasculitis. The vessels primarily involved in cutaneous vasculitis are the postcapillary venules, though capillaries and arterioles may also be inflamed. Often occurring as a result of hypersensitivity, a leucocytoclastic (necrotizing) appearance is seen on microscopy. The most common agents implicated in the pathogenesis of the disease are listed here.

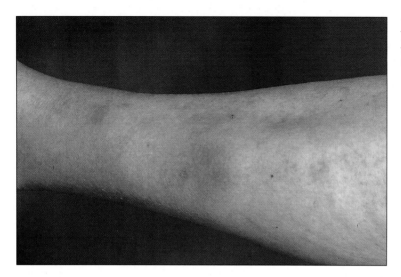

10.24 Mycoplasma vasculitis.
This young woman has a cutaneous vasculitis following infection with mycoplasma.

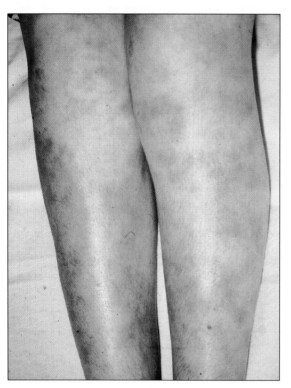

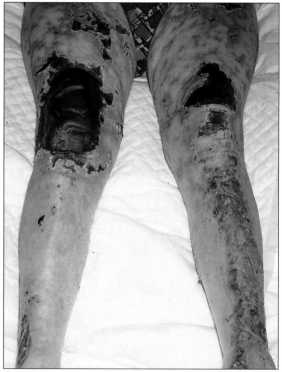

10.25 Erythema nodosum. Shown here in response to sulphonamide therapy, erythema nodosum is also vasculitic in nature. Initially presenting with painful erythematous nodules, the lesions resolve by mimicking the blue–brown discoloration of ecchymosis.

10.26 Cryoglobulins. These immune globulins in the serum precipitate or gel in the cold. They are found in small amounts in many 'normal' individuals and in increased amounts in a variety of diseases including infections, connective tissue diseases and lymphoproliferative disorders. A cutaneous vasculitis may coexist, as in this case, where cold precipitated the globulins in the cutaneous circulation, and vasculitis added to the ischaemic insult. These lesions, however, were superficial and healed with immunosuppressive therapy without the need for grafting.

11.

Visceral Arterial Disease

The main abdominal branches of the aorta are the coeliac artery, the superior mesenteric artery, the renal arteries and the inferior mesenteric artery. All of these arteries may become involved with disease, but in most cases this disease is effectively asymptomatic and it is only in a small number of cases that intervention is required. In addition, patients who have visceral arterial disease (including renal arterial disease) tend to have very severe generalized atherosclerosis that usually makes them unattractive candidates for major surgery.

Mesenteric ischaemia may be either acute, acute-on-chronic or chronic. In general, unless there is an acute thrombosis or embolus, two of the three main intestinal arteries must be severely compromised before intestinal ischaemia is likely. Clinical features of chronic disease include weight loss, fear of eating, severe postprandial pain and evidence of peripheral vascular disease.

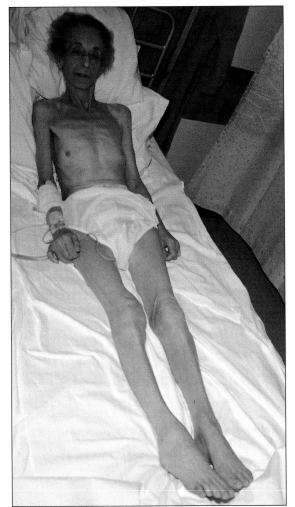

11.1 Emaciation in intestinal ischaemia. This woman had a 6-month history of severe abdominal pain with a normal gastroscopy and a normal barium enema and was eventually admitted to hospital with acute intractable abdominal pain. Laparoscopy revealed a very ischaemic bowel and she proceeded to angiography, which showed almost no visible mesenteric circulation.

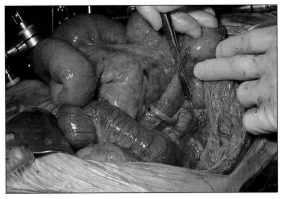

11.2 Aorto–mesenteric–coeliac bypass. At operation the coeliac and superior mesenteric arteries were occluded proximally, but found to have distal lumina. A vein bypass was therefore taken from the infrarenal aorta and passed retrojejunally up to the superior mesenteric artery.

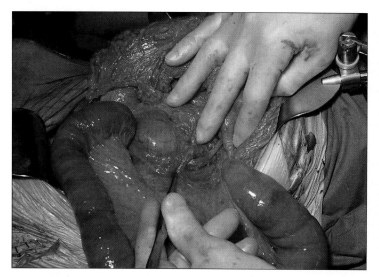

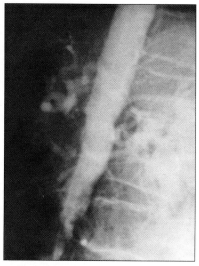

11.3 Aorto–mesenteric–coeliac bypass. This bypass was subsequently anastomosed side-to-side to the superior mesenteric artery and end-to-end to the coeliac artery. The ischaemic loops of small bowel can be easily seen here. Postoperatively the patient's pain disappeared immediately and at 3 months she had put on 15 kg of weight!

11.4 Coeliac artery occlusion. In this patient, angiography revealed an occluded coeliac artery with severe aortic atherosclerosis. The superior mesenteric artery was not visualized.

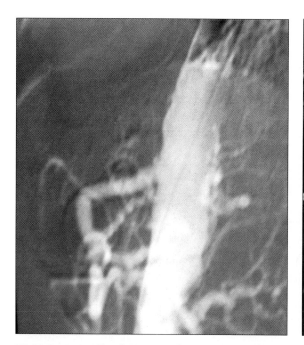

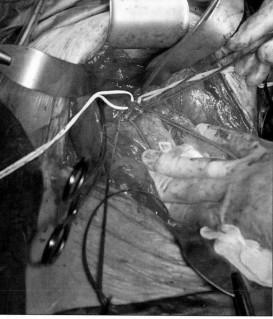

11.5 Aorto–coeliac bypass. In this case, the superior mesenteric artery was completely occluded throughout and the coeliac artery occluded at its origin. A single PTFE graft was therefore placed from the supracoeliac aorta to the coeliac trunk. The postoperative angiogram shows that this is a little too long. However, it is functioning well and the patient's symptoms were resolved at 6-month follow-up.

11.6 Coeliac artery exposure. The suprarenal aorta can be difficult to expose, but the operation is greatly facilitated by an abdominal wall retraction system such as the 'Omnitract' seen here. The coeliac trunk and its branches are dissected out before inserting a bifurcation graft into the supracoeliac aorta.

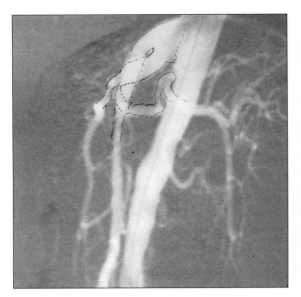

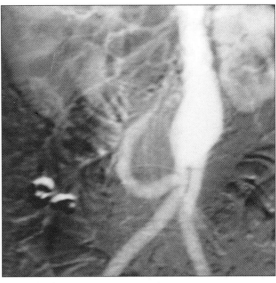

11.7 Aorto–coeliac/superior mesenteric artery bypass. Postoperative angiography shows the bypass graft in position and flow running into the coeliac and superior mesenteric arteries. This is a very effective bypass, but is technically a little more difficult to perform.

11.8 Aortic graft–superior mesenteric bypass. In this case, the patient was undergoing an aorto–bifemoral bypass for critical ischaemia, but was found to have a very ischaemic bowel. At operation, a side-graft was taken to the mesenteric artery and postoperative angiography showed the bypass to be functioning satisfactorily.

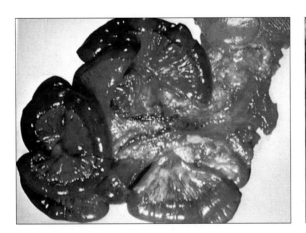

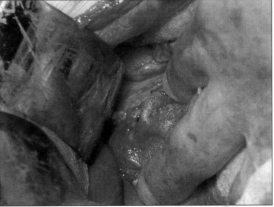

11.9 Acute arterial thrombosis or embolus. This may produce widespread gangrene of the intestine. Clinical features include sudden abdominal pain, minimal tenderness and a high white cell count. A high index of suspicion is required because without an early operation, the prognosis is dismal.

11.10 Coeliac artery compression. This is a somewhat doubtful entity in which abdominal pain is related to the compression of the coeliac axis by a tight band of tissue. The median arcuate ligament appears to be compressing the coeliac artery here, but releasing the band did not relieve the symptoms. It is highly unlikely that abdominal pain is ischaemic in origin when there are at least two normal mesenteric arteries.

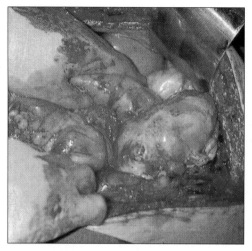

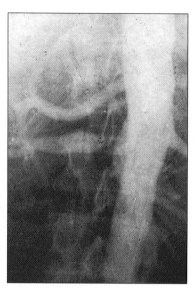

11.11 Sigmoid colon gangrene. Division of the inferior mesenteric artery is routine during abdominal aortic aneurysm surgery. Occasionally severe colonic ischaemia supervenes and a gangrenous sigmoid colon results. This may be avoided if a large 'meandering' collateral blood supply is seen and the inferior mesenteric artery is reimplanted or a bypass is performed to the superior mesenteric artery.

11.12 Renal artery stenosis. This is usually due to atherosclerosis, but in younger patients may be secondary to fibromuscular hyperplasia. Patients with unilateral stenosis may present with hypertension, but will not develop renal failure unless there is an underlying nephropathy or the other kidney also becomes involved. Treatment is therefore usually conservative with antihypertensives.

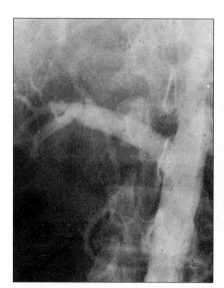

11.13 Surgical treatment of renal artery stenosis. Occasionally surgery is offered for renal artery stenosis, but this should be reserved for patients with renal failure. The treatment of hypertension with either renal artery surgery or angioplasty is disappointing with only about one-third of patients deriving any sustained benefit. Given the morbidity and potential mortality of these procedures, it is difficult to justify surgical intervention for hypertension alone.

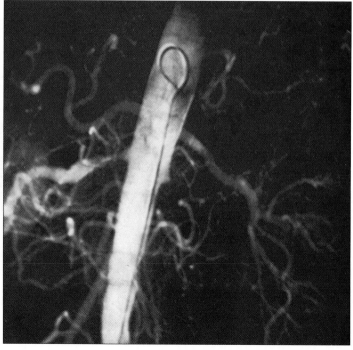

11.14 Left spleno–renal artery bypass. Extra-anatomic revascularization of the left renal artery has been performed by joining the splenic artery to the transected left renal artery as an end-to-end anastomosis. This can be carried out with minimum morbidity in patients in whom aortic clamping is inadvisable.

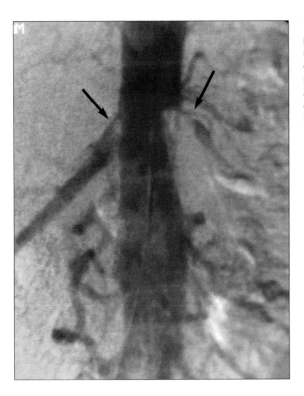

11.15 Severe bilateral renal artery stenosis. This patient had severe atherosclerotic disease of the aorta and renal arteries (arrows) associated with chronic renal failure and hypertension. He also had severe cardiac disease that precluded any consideration of surgery for his condition. Many patients with end-stage renal artery disease have coexistent medical conditions that prevent surgical intervention or make it extremely risky.

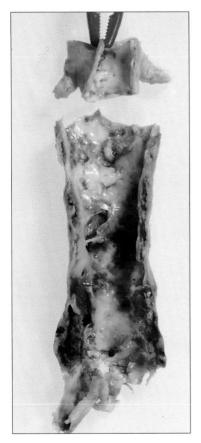

11.16 Aorto–renal endarterectomy. In some instances, it is possible to revascularize both renal arteries simultaneously by performing an endarterectomy. This specimen, which was retrieved after aorto–renal endarterectomy, shows the perirenal endarterectomy separate from the main piece. In these cases, a supracoeliac clamp is temporarily placed until the renal stage is complete. The aortic clamp is then repositioned to an infrarenal level allowing the rest of the operation to be completed at a more leisurely pace.

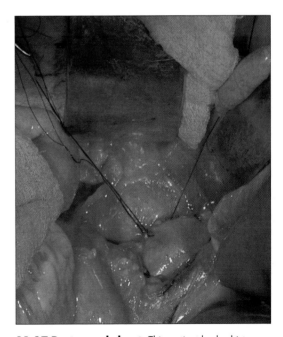

11.17 Portacaval shunt. This patient had a history of longstanding cirrhosis and portal hypertension with oesophageal variceal bleeds. It was eventually decided to treat him with a portasystemic shunt and here the shunt may be seen after completion (side-to-side).

12.

Tumours of Blood Vessels

Haemangioma is the term used to describe a tumour of the superficial (usually skin) blood vessel. Haemangiomas include capillary haemangiomas (e.g. port-wine stain, strawberry mark) and cavernous haemangiomas.

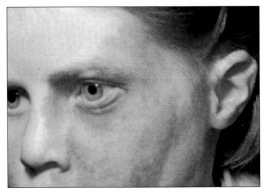

12.1 Capillary haemangioma. The port-wine stain is a flat slow-growing capillary haemangioma. It does not regress, but may require excision and skin graft. More novel treatments of this 'birthmark' include tattooing with skin-coloured material and laser removal.

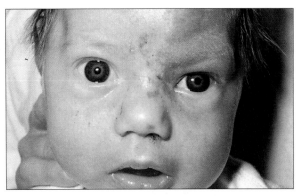

12.2 Haemangioma. This may be associated with similar lesions in neural tissue. The Sturge–Weber syndrome shown here comprises a port-wine stain in addition to a capillary haemangioma in the meninges and the choroid coat of the eye.

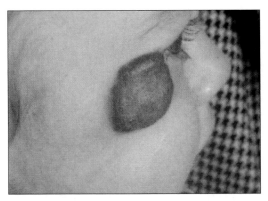

12.3 The raised or strawberry naevus. This appears shortly after birth, grows slowly for months, and disappears after a few years. No treatment is therefore required.

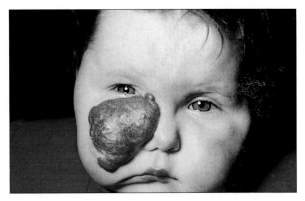

12.4 The cavernous haemangioma. This soft, easily compressible lesion may occur in subcutaneous or submucous areas as well as in the viscera. It is composed of large irregular blood spaces.

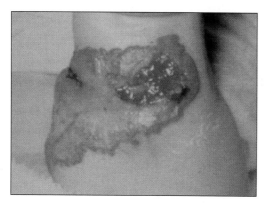

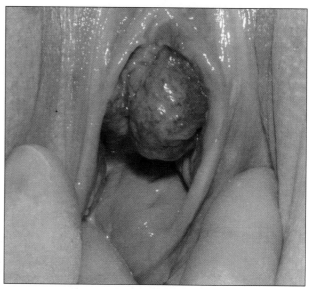

12.5 Cavernous haemangioma. Complications that can be serious include ulceration, bleeding and infection.

12.6 Cavernous haemangioma. This was noted in the vagina in a pregnant woman. It became larger with pregnancy and was removed because it was feared that it might endanger labour.

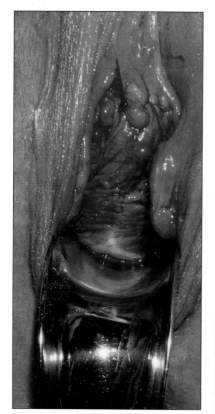

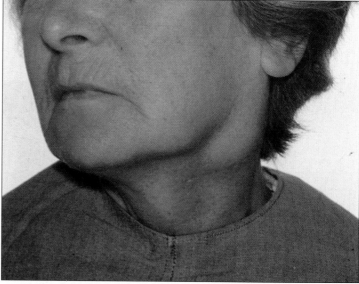

12.7 The haemangioma in 12.6 was easily excised. Labour progressed without problems.

12.8 Carotid body tumour. This appears as a symptomless, often longstanding, swelling at the angle of the jaw where it may be mistaken for a parotid tumour or enlarged lymph gland. It is mobile from side to side, but not vertically.

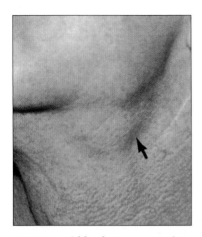

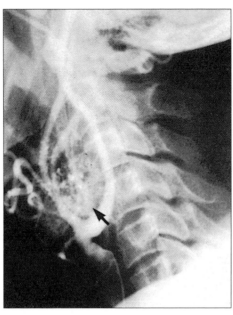

12.9 Carotid body tumour. In this patient the tumour was much smaller than in **12.8** and a little anterior to the angle of the jaw. The level was similar—at the bifurcation of the carotid artery.

12.10 Chemodectoma. A carotid body tumour is really a chemodectoma and not a tumour of blood vessels, but it is vascular and very clearly associated with the carotid arteries. Angiography shows the separation of the carotid vessels by the tumour (goblet displacement) and the blush of vessels in the tumour.

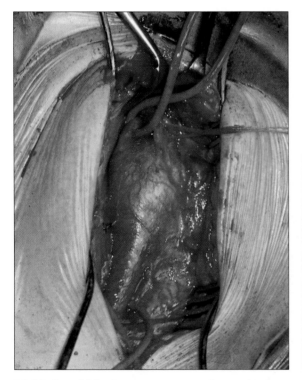

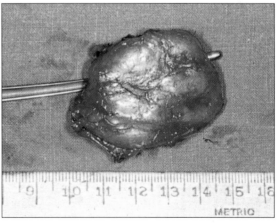

12.11 Carotid body tumour exposed at operation. The internal carotid artery has a rubber string around it. The tumour arose from the undersurface of the carotid bifurcation, to which it was closely adherent. Growth occurs upwards. A transmitted pulsation and a bruit were present, but not expansile pulsation. The hypoglossal nerve was close to the upper end of the tumour.

12.12 An excised carotid body tumour. The tumour was well encapsulated. The probe was passed through the external carotid artery, which was so involved that its resection made the operation easier.

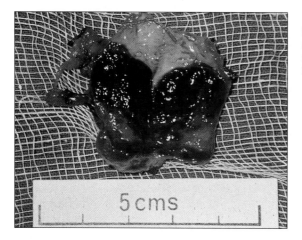

12.13 Incised carotid body tumour. The cut surface of the tumour gives an idea of its vascularity. The tumour may show histological evidence of malignancy, but its growth is usually very slow so resection is not always mandatory. Local invasion is more common than distant metastases.

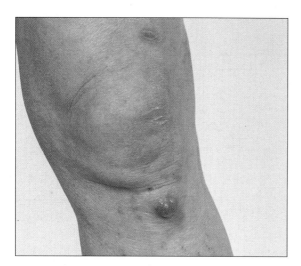

12.14 A glomangioma (glomus tumour). This presented as a painful red–blue swelling in the skin of the limb. In this case the swelling below the knee was well localized and curiously tender. It may appear under the nails, especially in females.

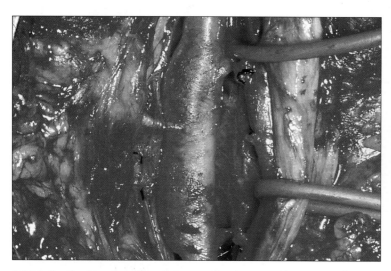

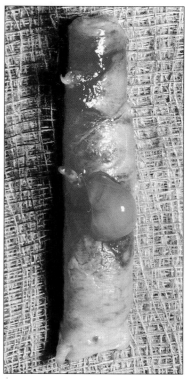

12.15 Cystic degeneration of the popliteal artery. This is not really a tumour of blood vessels. However, the condition is a mucoid cyst of the adventitia in the middle third of the artery. It produces a narrowing of the vessel with claudication. The area is seen at operation as a bulge.

12.16 Excised cystic area of the popliteal artery. The cystic area is excised *in toto* and a graft inserted. The mucoid nature of the lesion is evident.

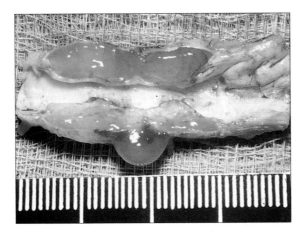

12.17 Popliteal stenosis. The mucocystic condition is even more evident when the lesion is opened up. The area of popliteal stenosis is clearly seen.

MALIGNANT TUMOURS OF BLOOD VESSELS

These are rather rare and include angiosarcoma and Kaposi's sarcoma. Kaposi's sarcoma is becoming more common with the development of these tumours in patients suffering from AIDS.

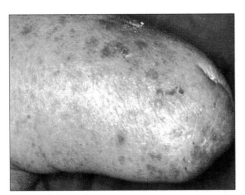

12.18 Kaposi's sarcoma. This was previously more commonly seen in equatorial Africa than in Europe. It appears as nodular lesions that are a purple or brown colour. In this case the lesions appeared on an amputation stump. Biopsy establishes the diagnosis.

13.

Arteriovenous Fistulae

An arteriovenous fistula is an abnormal connection between an artery and vein. Such fistulae may be congenital (multiple or localized) or acquired.

CONGENITAL ARTERIOVENOUS FISTULAE

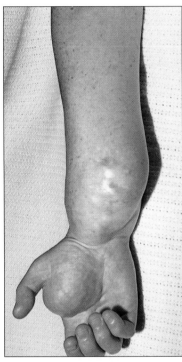

13.1 Arteriovenous fistula. Here, this involves the radial artery in a 40-year-old woman. Two swellings are present—one in the forearm, the other in the hand. The scar of a previous surgical attempt at closure can be seen. The fistulae were multiple, but there was no overgrowth of the arm or hand. A soft bruit was heard.

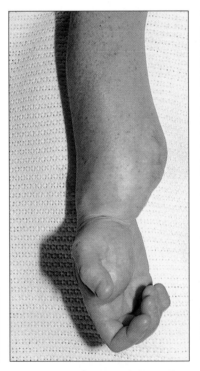

13.2 A lateral view of 13.1. This shows the marked swelling. Movement of the thumb and index finger was limited, but was less limited in the other fingers. At a second operation the dilated veins contained a considerable amount of blood clot.

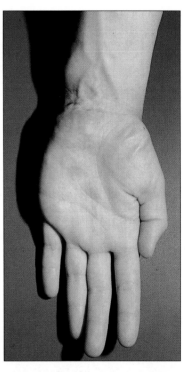

13.3 Localized arteriovenous fistula. This was a more localized arteriovenous fistula in a teenage girl, affecting the hypothenar eminence. The proximal veins are prominent. A thrill was noticeable and a murmur was clearly heard.

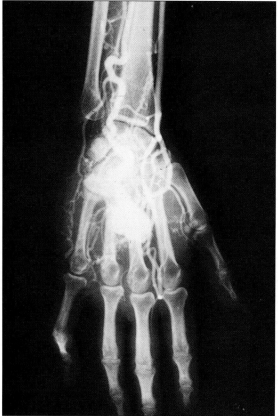

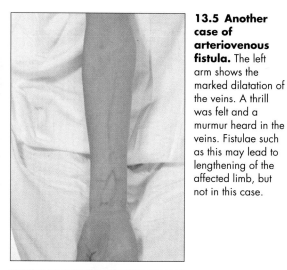

13.5 Another case of arteriovenous fistula. The left arm shows the marked dilatation of the veins. A thrill was felt and a murmur heard in the veins. Fistulae such as this may lead to lengthening of the affected limb, but not in this case.

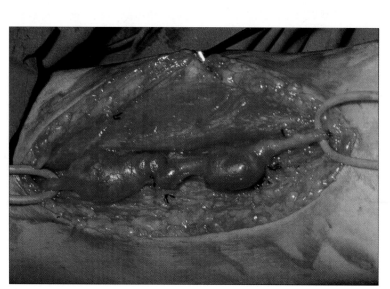

13.4 Localized arteriovenous fistula. The angiogram showed a mass of vessels in the hypothenar area. A dilated vein is shown passing up the arm close to the ulnar artery. At operation a fistula was demonstrated between the ulnar artery and vein. Closure of this relieved the patient's complaint.

13.6 Multiple aneurysms. A curious feature of the case described in **13.5** was the presence of multiple aneurysms of the brachial artery. These were saccular and presumably related to a congenital weakness in the muscular wall of the artery.

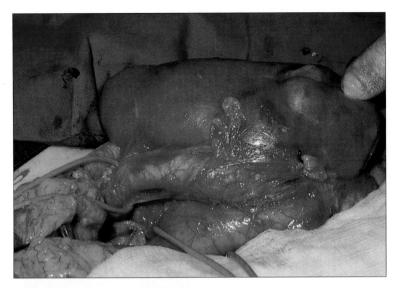

13.7 Congenital arteriovenous fistula. This may occur in any part of the body. This patient, a 40-year-old woman, presented with haematuria. Arteriography demonstrated a fistula, which was found at operation to be between the renal artery and a very large renal vein, shown with the rubber around it in the lower part of the picture.

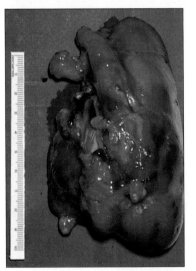

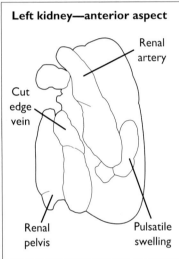

Left kidney—anterior aspect

Renal artery

Cut edge vein

Renal pelvis

Pulsatile swelling

13.8 Fistula between renal artery and renal vein. The kidney and fistula described in **13.7** are shown along with a diagram of the fistula.

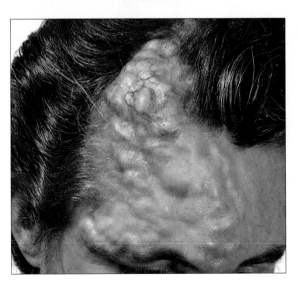

13.9 Cirsoid aneurysm. This complicated arteriovenous fistula involving the superficial temporal artery and vein, with a connection with the cerebral vessels, occurred in this man's teens. It is sometimes termed a 'cirsoid aneurysm'. There was a marked thrill and bruit. Ligation of the right external carotid artery markedly improved the situation, but further surgery with excision of the vessels was necessary.

ACQUIRED ARTERIOVENOUS FISTULAE

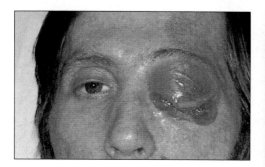

13.10 Carotid–cavernous fistula. This may follow a skull fracture or the rupture of an arterial aneurysm into a vein. The latter was thought to be the case in this man. It produced the classic, if rare, sign of a pulsating exophthalmos.

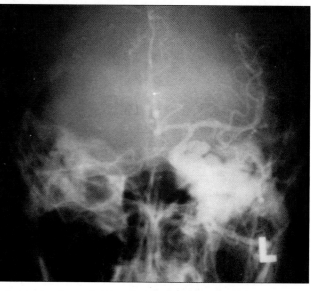

13.11 Fistula and dilated vessels. An angiogram showed the area of the fistula and the dilated vessels draining it.

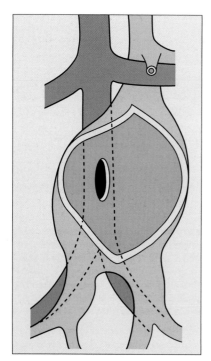

13.12 Ruptured aortic aneurysm. Rarely, an abdominal aortic aneurysm may rupture into the inferior vena cava. The drawing represents the findings at an emergency operation for resection of a ruptured aortic aneurysm. A marked thrill was palpable in the inferior vena cava at operation.

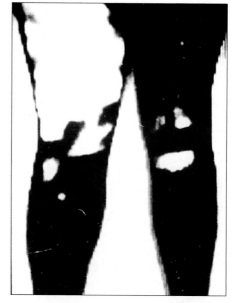

13.13 Traumatic arteriovenous fistula. Thermography may illustrate the area of increased vascularity in association with an arteriovenous fistula. The white area in the right thigh is the site of a traumatic arteriovenous fistula, the development of which followed a knife wound.

14.

Venous Disease

CONGENITAL ABNORMALITIES

Congenital abnormalities are rare. They can be broadly classified into two groups: angiomata of veins (phlebangioma) and dilated venous trunks (phlebectasia). More common are arteriovenous fistulae in which the dilated veins are a secondary response to increased flow due to an abnormal arterial–venous connection.

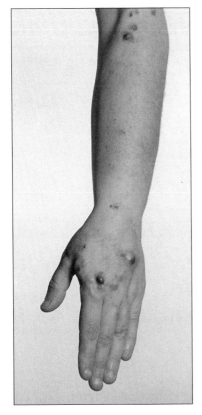

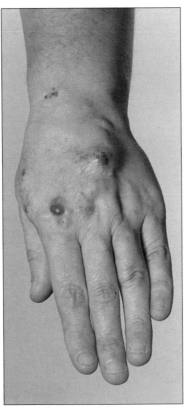

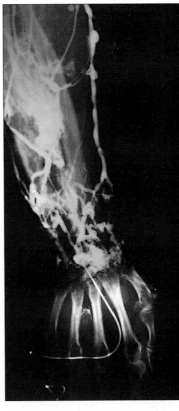

14.1 Phlebectasia. This had been present in the arm of this middle-aged woman since childhood. Within the dilated veins there was evidence of thrombosis and areas of thrombosis calcification may develop, which can be seen as white flecks on plain radiography.

14.2 Phlebangioma. This is easily seen if on the dorsum of the hand, as here.

14.3 Venography of the arm. This demonstrates the dilated veins with saccular areas, and the collection of phlebangiomas at the wrist.

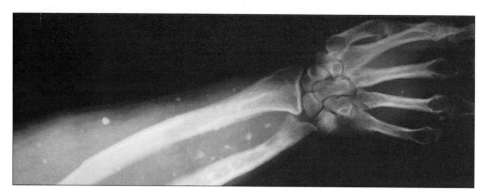

14.4 Calcification within areas of longstanding thrombosis. These are easily visible on a plain radiograph.

VARICOSE VEINS

Varicose veins are dilated tortuous superficial veins of the leg. They result when a raised intraluminal pressure is abnormally transmitted from the deep to the superficial veins due to a failure of the valvular mechanism, which normally prevents this transmission. Varicose veins can be either primary if there is no preceding pathological cause, or secondary, in which case there is a preceding cause (e.g. deep vein thrombosis).

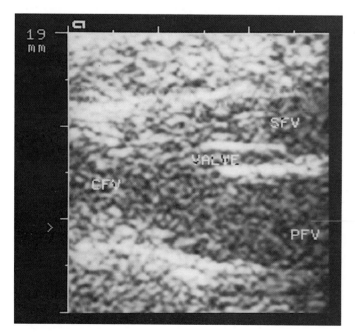

14.5 B-mode ultrasound. A superficial femoral vein valve is shown.

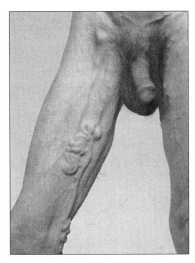

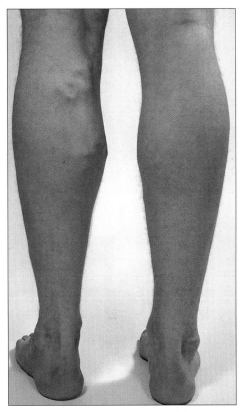

14.7 Primary varicose veins of the short saphenous system.

Approximately 10% of varicose veins are primary varicose veins of the short saphenous system and may occur with or without varicose veins of the long saphenous vein. Most veins on the posterior surface of the calf are due to a tributary of the long saphenous system rather than of the short saphenous system.

14.6 Primary varicose veins of the long saphenous distribution.

These can be seen originating from the groin and passing down the medial aspect of the leg. There is also a varicocoele at the groin. This is a gross, usually saccular, dilatation of the origin of the long saphenous vein. The tortuous nature of varicose veins is well demonstrated, particularly in the mid thigh.

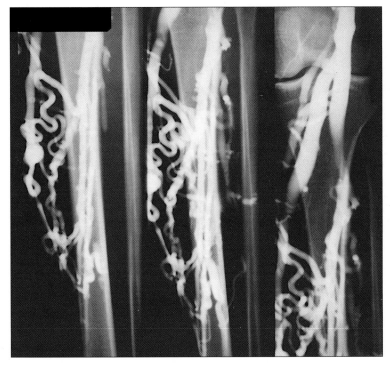

14.8 Varicography.
Contrast is directly injected into a varicosity to demonstrate the connection between the deep and superficial systems. In this case the short saphenous vein is responsible.

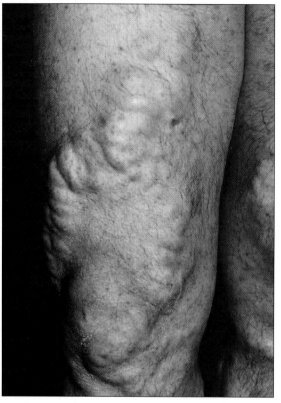

14.9 Primary varicose veins. These may become grossly dilated and contain a relatively large volume of blood. In this case the dilatation is of the medial tributary of the long saphenous vein.

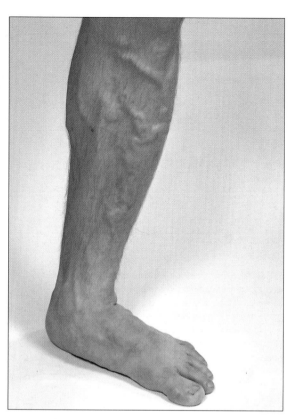

14.10 Primary varicose veins. The varicose veins may also arise solely from a perforator connecting the deep and superficial systems below the level of the groin and the sapheno–femoral junction.

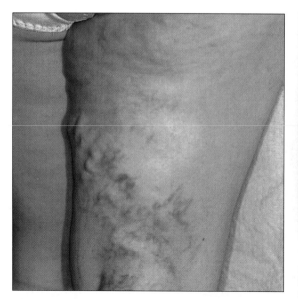

14.11 Varicose veins arising in the posterior thigh. These are often derived directly from the profunda femoris vein.

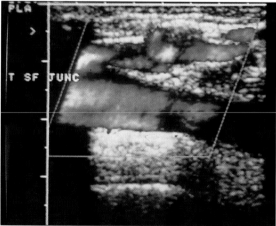

14.12 Duplex scanning of varicose veins. A noninvasive method of visualizing both the anatomy and function within veins, duplex is a combination of normal B-mode ultrasound and directional Doppler in which a Doppler signal can be obtained from structures visualized on the ultrasound picture. In the case shown proximal flow is to the left and is assigned a blue colour.

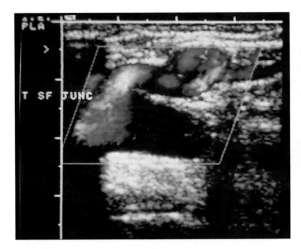

14.13 Reverse flow within veins. This is only possible when the unidirectional valvular mechanism is lost. This is represented by the change in colour to red (i.e. flow to the right).

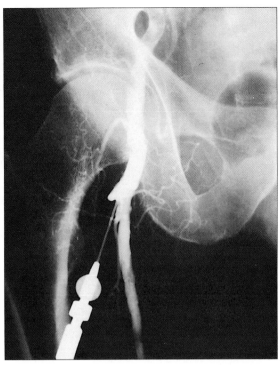

14.14 Venography. Here, venography by direct groin puncture fails to show any reflux from the deep system (common femoral vein) to the superficial system (long saphenous vein). This illustrates the competency of the valve at the sapheno–femoral junction.

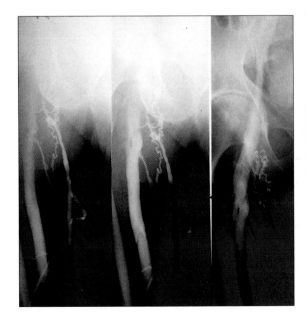

14.15 Varicography. The investigation of choice for recurrent varicose veins is varicography. In two-thirds of patients the recurrence is due to an inadequate primary groin operation, which fails to disconnect the superficial and deep systems.

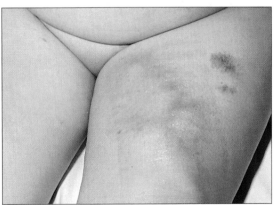

14.16 Superficial thrombophlebitis. A well-recognized complication of varicose veins is superficial thrombophlebitis. The inflammation may be associated with complete thrombosis of the vein and may rarely propagate to the deep veins. In the example shown the veins affected can be clearly seen and are on the anterior thigh.

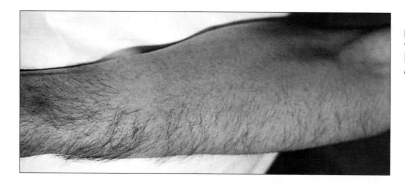

14.17 Superficial thrombophlebitis. This can occur without varicose veins, as in this patient who had an intravenous infusion into the arm.

CHRONIC VENOUS INSUFFICIENCY

Chronic venous insufficiency is the result of sustained venous hypertension. It may result from venous reflux due to either superficial or deep vein valve failure/ incompetence or outflow obstruction (e.g. post deep vein thrombosis), or a combination of both.

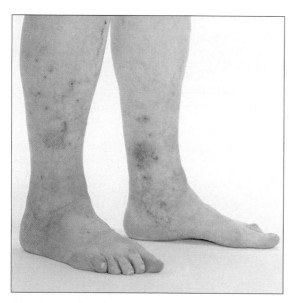

14.18 Acute lipodermatosclerosis. Findings of early chronic venous insufficiency may include acute lipodermatosclerosis, which is seen in the gaiter area above the malleoli. It is an acute inflammatory response of lipodermatosclerosis and is often indistinguishable from acute cellulitis. There is some evidence that a component of this inflammatory response is due to proliferation of skin capillaries.

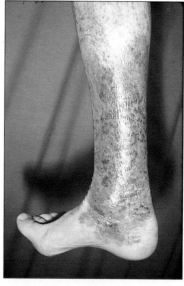

14.19 Eczema/dermatitis. This may be present, particularly in the medial supramalleolar area, and may be due to chronic venous insufficiency (varicose eczema) or be an allergic response to local therapy.

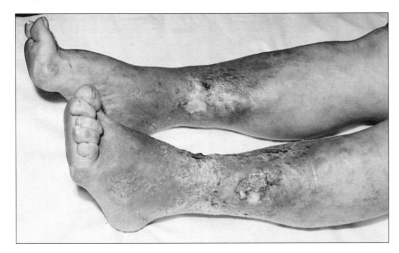

14.20 Lipodermatosclerosis. This occurs with more longstanding chronic venous insufficiency. It is a combination of fat necrosis, chronic inflammatory induration and scarring. There is also a characteristic brown pigmentation and, occasionally, calcification.

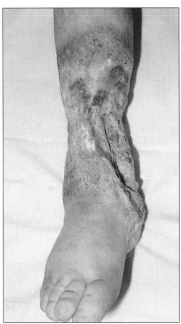

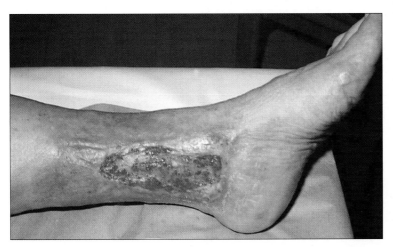

14.21 Leg ulceration. In this case the ulceration is in the classic supramedial malleolar position (or gaiter area). There is also a surrounding area of varicose eczema.

14.22 Leg ulceration. This may be more extensive, but can still be seen to be essentially perimalleolar. Venous ulceration is characterized by its cyclical nature of healing and breakdown. In the case shown here there is also foot oedema, which is probably due to lymphatic channel fibrosis as a consequence of recurrent infection.

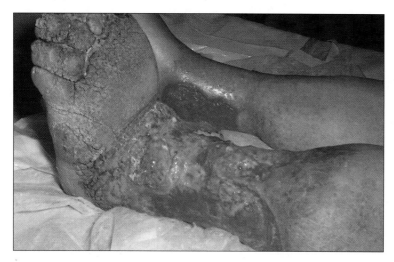

14.23 Leg ulceration. This may become circumferential (right leg), causing an 'elephant's foot' appearance. This is produced by lymphoedema due to lymphatic fibrosis caused by recurrent lymphangitis, which is in turn secondary to repeated cellulitis. There is an element of local lymphatic damage secondary to the presence of such a large circumferential ulcer.

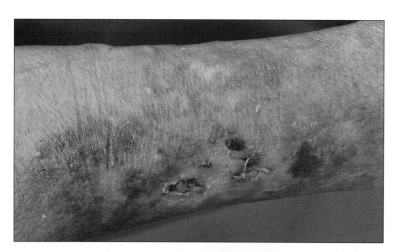

14.24 Calcification. This can be palpated in some legs with chronic venous ulceration. As previously mentioned it is due to calcification of thrombus within superficial varicosities.

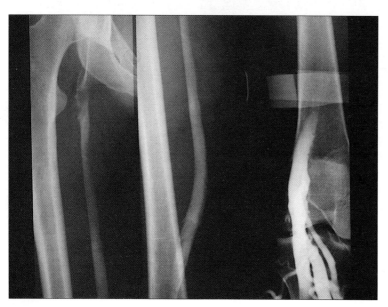

14.25 Incompetent deep valves. These may be the cause of chronic venous insufficiency. Postphlebitic changes can also be responsible due to secondary deep venous obstruction and/or valvular incompetence. In the example shown there is no evidence for deep venous scarring and this is therefore a case of primary deep valve failure.

DEEP VEIN THROMBOSIS

Deep vein thrombosis (DVT) is a relatively common clinical problem, but the true incidence is difficult to assess. The common symptoms and signs are local tenderness, local erythema, increased local temperature, local swelling and dilated superficial veins.

The pathophysiological factors are categorized according to Virchow's triad: an alteration in the vessel wall, changes in blood coagulability and a modification in blood flow.

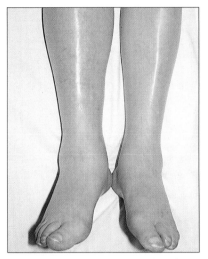

14.26 Phlegmasia alba dolens. This is typically due to an acute oedema of the leg as a result of an isolated iliofemoral vein thrombosis with an associated lymphatic obstruction.

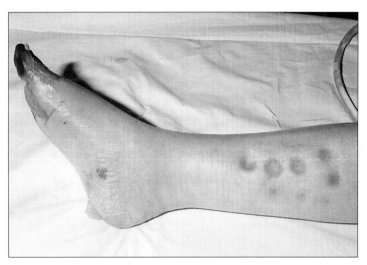

14.27 Pitting oedema. This is demonstrated in most cases of acute deep vein thrombosis, but particularly with phlegmasia alba dolens.

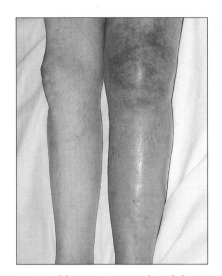

14.28 Phlegmasia caerulea dolens. This involves more extensive thrombosis in the venous drainage of the leg, which leads to intense swelling. Eventually the increasing venous outflow obstruction impedes arterial inflow.

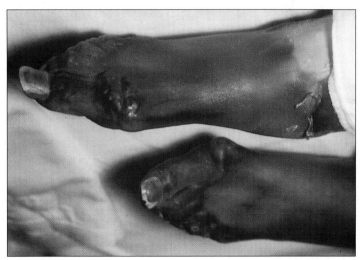

14.29 Venous gangrene. This is the result of inflow failure due to venous outflow obstruction. It is associated with poor demarcation, gross swelling and toxaemia.

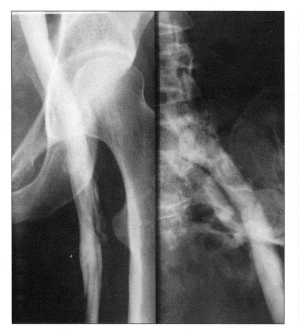

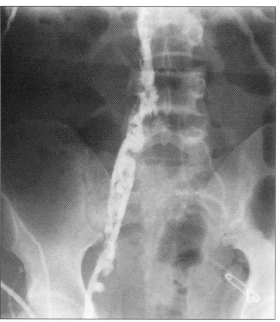

14.30 Venography. The 'gold standard' for the diagnosis of DVT is venography. However, it is uncomfortable and carries the risks associated with radiographic contrast and the risk of causing DVT. In the example shown here there is a smooth flow of the contrast with no filling defects.

14.31 Venography. In this case venography demonstrates thrombus within the iliac system extending into the inferior vena cava.

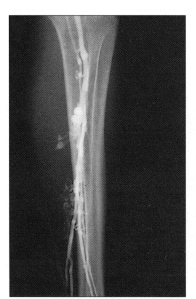

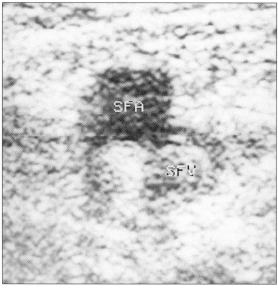

14.32 Venography. This shows a DVT affecting the calf vessels.

14.33 Duplex scan. This noninvasive method of diagnosing DVT is now regarded as the first line of investigation. In this case the thrombus can be seen within the vein; this has the effect of reducing flow through the segment and renders the vein relatively incompressible.

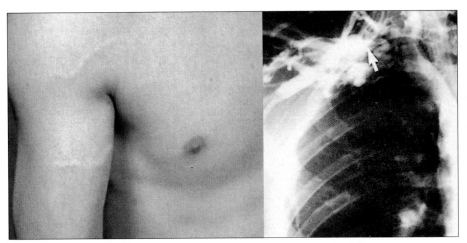

14.34 Axillary vein thrombosis. This may also occur. Distended upper arm veins can be seen in the clinical photograph shown here. The venogram shows blockage of the axillary vein (arrow).

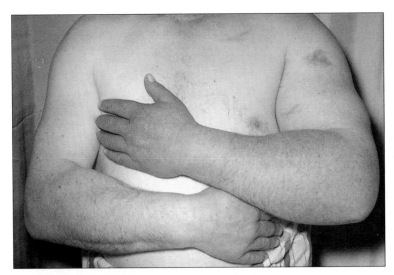

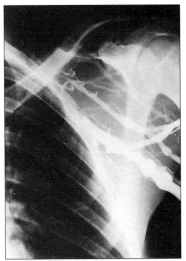

14.35 Axillary/subclavian vein thrombosis. This is less common. In the case shown here, the left arm of a 56-year-old man is swollen with a bluish tinge. Following both axillary and subclavian vein thrombosis, the patient may unfortunately not return to full function.

14.36 Venography. This shows extensive blockage of the axillary vein of the patient in **14.35**. The precise aetiology of this case is unknown, but the patient had been painting the ceiling prior to admission, and a degree of cervical outlet compression may have played a role.

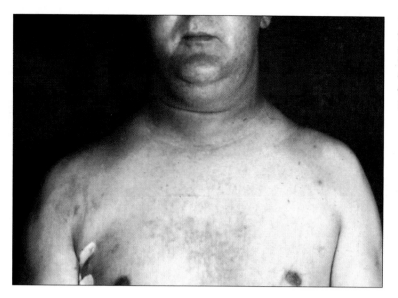

14.37 Superior vena caval thrombosis. This condition is usually associated with tumour compression of the vessel. It produces a bluish-red discoloration and swelling of the upper chest and neck with prominent permanently filling veins.

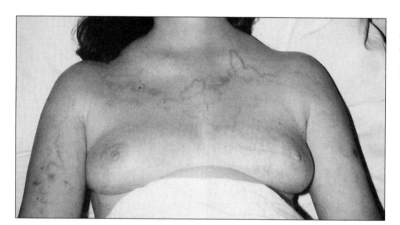

14.38 Superior vena caval thrombosis. In this woman superior vena caval thrombosis has resulted in a network of prominent veins across the upper chest and both arms.

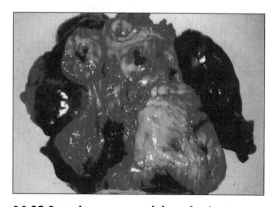

14.39 Superior vena caval thrombosis. A postmortem specimen showing malignant glands surrounding the vessel and producing compression and eventual thrombosis. The opening of the subclavian vein can be seen, with clot in the lower part of the superior vena cava.

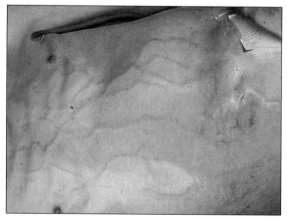

14.40 Inferior vena caval thrombosis. This is also associated with malignant disease. There are distended abdominal and lower chest veins accompanied by oedema of the legs.

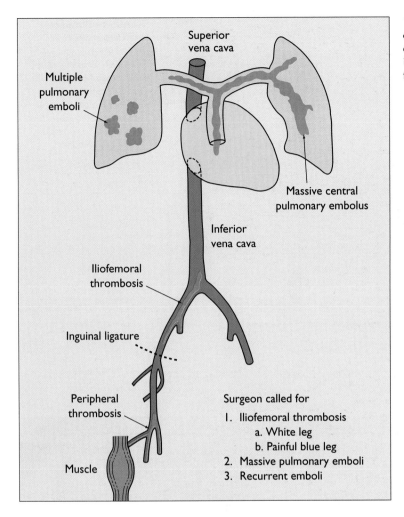

14.41 Thromboembolism. This is due to thrombus within veins embolising to the lungs. This diagram illustrates the sites of thrombosis and the types of pulmonary embolism.

Superior vena cava

Multiple pulmonary emboli

Massive central pulmonary embolus

Inferior vena cava

Iliofemoral thrombosis

Inguinal ligature

Peripheral thrombosis

Muscle

Surgeon called for

1. Iliofemoral thrombosis
     a. White leg
     b. Painful blue leg
2. Massive pulmonary emboli
3. Recurrent emboli

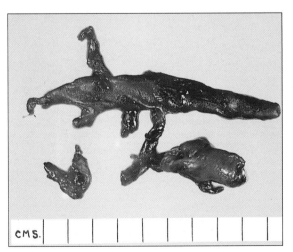

CMS.

14.42 Pulmonary embolus (PE). Manifestations of a PE range from sudden death, to collapse and hypotension, to breathlessness and chest pain with blood-stained sputum, to tachypnoea. Multiple episodes of PE may produce pulmonary hypertension. The emboli shown here were removed by emergency pulmonary artery thrombectomy.

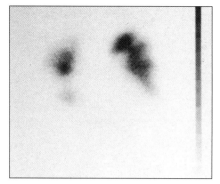

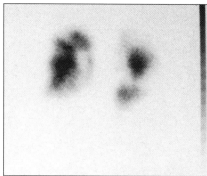

14.43 Ventilation/ perfusion scan. This may lead to the diagnosis of pulmonary embolus. In the case shown here multiple perfusion defects, which were not matched by the ventilation scan, mean that the diagnosis is probably pulmonary embolism.

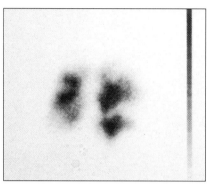

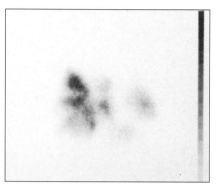

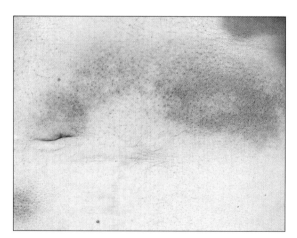

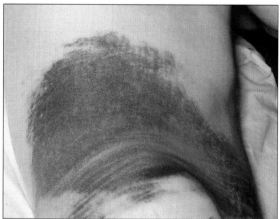

14.44 Subcutaneous heparin. One of the standard measures to prevent DVT or pulmonary embolus is subcutaneous heparin administration, but this can produce bruising of the injection site, as shown here.

14.45 Anticoagulation. The standard method of treatment of venous thromboembolism is anticoagulation; however, a lack of care in controlling the degree of anticoagulation can produce haemorrhagic complications, as in this patient with a large retroperitoneal bleed.

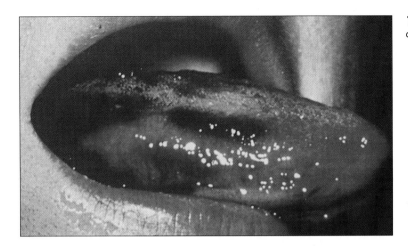

14.46 Glossal haematoma. This is a consequence of over-anticoagulation.

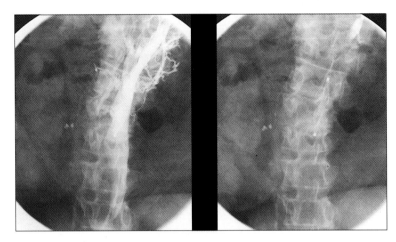

14.47 Vena caval filter. This should be considered in the management of pulmonary embolus if there is a strong contraindication to anticoagulation, if there are recurrent pulmonary emboli despite adequate anticoagulation, or if an ascending venogram reveals that the morphology of the clot indicates a high risk of massive pulmonary embolus (i.e. intracaval or free clot).

15.

Lymphoedema of the Lower Limb

The lymphatic system is responsible for the transporting tissue fluid—lymph (cells, protein and water)—from the intercellular space to the blood stream. It comprises a network of lymph capillaries and vessels, the lymph nodes, and aggregations of lymph tissues in the spleen and thymus and around the alimentary tract. The direction of lymph flow is controlled by the presence of valves within lymph vessels.

Lymphoedema is the swelling of a body part due to an abnormal intercellular build-up of water and protein as a consequence of a disorder in the lymphatic transport system. Lymphoedema can be classified into primary and secondary lymphoedema. In turn, primary lymphoedema can subdivided in two ways.

- By age of presentation: congenital (present at birth, 10%); praecox (starting before 35 years of age); tarda (starting at 35 years of age). When lymphoedema is congenital and familial (autosomal dominant), it is known as Milroy's disease (2% of all patients).
- By lympangiographic appearance: aplasia (no lymphatics seen); hypoplasia (fewer and smaller lymphatics than normal); hyperplasia (many more or very dilated lymphatics).

Secondary lymphoedema results from an identifiable cause, which may be one of the following:

- Malignant disease involving the lymphatic drainage (i.e. inguinal or axillary nodes).
- Surgery with dissection of the regional nodes (i.e. inguinal or axillary nodes).
- Radiation damage (particularly in conjunction with surgery).
- Infection: either recurrent pyogenic infection (staphylococcus or beta-haemolytic streptococci), particularly in cases of chronic venous ulceration; or in Africa or India due to *Wuchereria bancrofti* (filariasis), in which the parasite invades the lymphatic system and thereby obstructs it.

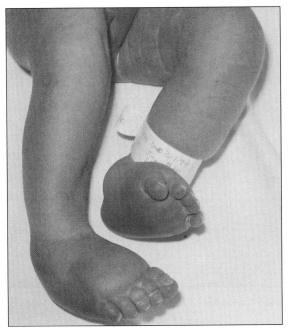

15.1 Primary lymphoedema. This case is in a neonate and is classified as congenital primary lymphoedema, which accounts for 10% of cases.

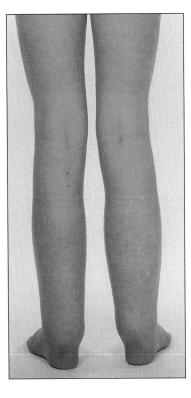

15.2 Primary lymphoedema. This 15-year-old boy with bilateral swollen legs presented at birth and had a strong family history (i.e. Milroy's disease).

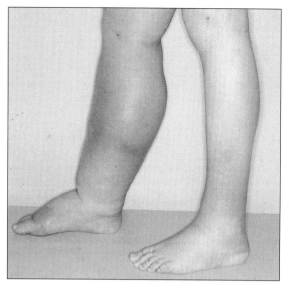

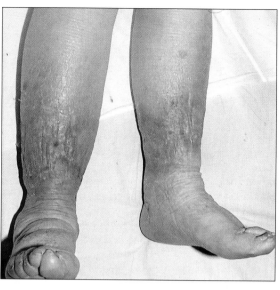

15.3 Primary lymphoedema. The condition may present as a unilateral leg swelling, but may eventually progress to become bilateral. Initially the oedema is soft and easily pitted; however, as time passes pitting may not be possible and the skin becomes progressively thicker and rougher. The contours of the leg are gradually lost and the limb adopts a 'tree trunk-like' configuration.

15.4 Primary lymphoedema. This 50-year-old female presented after 35 years of age (i.e. lymphoedema tarda) and now has an associated recurrent cellulitis leading to skin thickening and the classical 'peau d'orange' appearance.

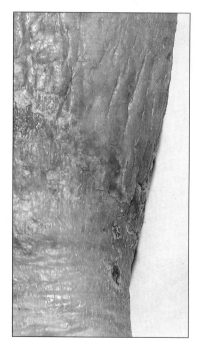

15.5 Primary lymphoedema. A close-up view of the patient in **15.4** shows evidence of hyperkeratosis and skin fissuring, the latter allowing bacterial entry and recurrent cellulitis. Treatment of infection is important in terms of comfort and preventing further infective lymphatic obliteration.

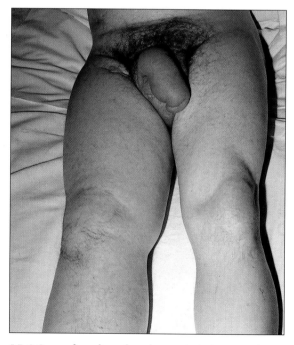

15.6 Secondary lymphoedema. As in this example, this may result from a malignant blockage of regional nodes, in this case in the right groin. This may be worsened by either surgery or radiotherapy. A 'bursting' pain may occur, but severe pain is unusual in lymphoedema and if present is likely to be due to nerve injury or malignant infiltration.

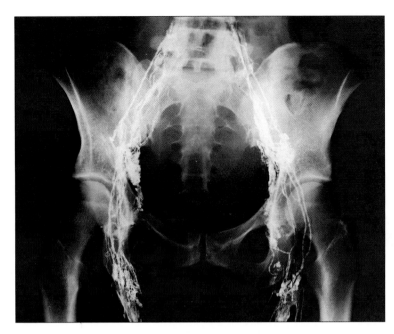

15.7 Lymphangiography. This should be reserved for those patients in whom it will make a therapeutic difference (i.e. patients with primary lymphoedema and suspected proximal obstruction or valvular incompetence). A normal lymphangiogram is shown, with numerous vessels streaming through normal lymph nodes.

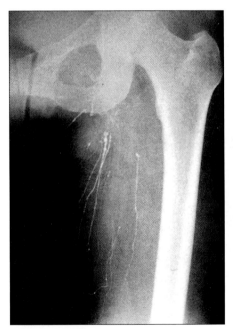

15.8 Hypoplastic lymphangiogram. Spidery and sparse lymphatic channels are shown.

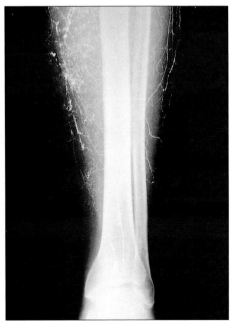

15.9 Hyperplastic lymphangiogram. The hyperplasia shown here is due to proximal nodal blockage rather than being part of a developmental abnormality.

TUMOUR OF THE LYMPHATIC SYSTEM

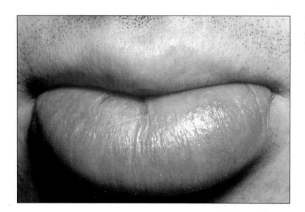

15.10 Lymphangioma. This benign tumour of lymphatic vessels is relatively uncommon, but in the case shown here has involved the lower lip, producing a macrocheilia.

TREATMENT OF LYMPHOEDEMA

Lymphoedema may be treated conservatively using compression stockings or pneumatic compression boots. Surgical treatment consists of either reducing operations, which consist of 'debulking' the affected limb, or bypass operations, in which an attempt is made to produce new lymphatic channels draining the limb.

Lymphoedema is a progressive condition and causes gradual enlarging of the limb.

Index

Note: numbers in normal type are page numbers, those in **bold** are **figure** numbers.